JONEEBA!

*The Exciting Workout and Fitness
Program with the Dances
and Drums of Africa*

JONEEBA!

The Exciting Workout and Fitness Program with the Dances and Drums of Africa

BY

A. DJONIBA MOUFLET

with Mali M. Fleming, Tyran Mincey, D.C., Certified Applied Kinesiologist, Lara Anasaze, M.S., Nutritionist & Exercise Physiologist, and Misani

SPECIAL PARTICIPATION OF ADRIENNE INGRUM

HATHERLEIGH PRESS

NEW YORK

A Getfitnow.com Book

JONEEBA! The Exciting Workout and Fitness Program
with the Dances and Drums of Africa
A Getfitnow.com Book

Hatherleigh Press/Getfitnow.com Books
An Affiliate of W.W. Norton & Company, Inc.
500 Fifth Ave
New York, NY 10110
1-800-367-2550

Visit our website: www.getfitnow.com

Disclaimer:
Before beginning any exercise program consult your physician. The author
and publisher of this book and workout disclaim any liability, personal or
professional, resulting from the misapplication of any of the training
procedures described in this publication.

All Getfitnow.com titles are available for bulk purchase, special promotions,
and premiums. For more information, please contact the manager of our
Special Sales Department at 1-800-367-2550.

Library of Congress Cataloging-in-Publication Data

    Mouflet, A. Djoniba, 1961-
        Joneeba!: The African dance workout / by A. Djoniba Mouflet with
        Mali Michelle Fleming and Misani; special participation of Adrienne
        Ingrum, Tyran, Mincey, and Lara Anasaze.
          p. cm.
        Includes bibliographical references and index.
        ISBN 1-57826-049-3 (alk. paper)
          1. Exercise. 2. Dance—Africa. I. Title: African dance workout.
        II. Fleming, Mali Michelle. III. Misani. IV. Title.
    GV481. M644 2000
    613.7'1—dc21   00-26779

Cover design by Lisa Fyfe
Text design and composition by DC Designs

Principal photography by Peter Field Peck with Canon® cameras and lenses
on Fuji® color negative film
Printed on acid-free paper
10 9 8 7 6 5 4 3 2 1

Additional photography in Senegal, West Africa, courtesy of Pap Ba.

African Dance is a Great Workout...

Take a **JONEEBA!** Class

As a Workout or a Cultural Journey.

HEAR THE RHYTHM...
LET THE DRUMS
FREE YOUR MIND
FOLLOW THE SPIRIT
IT'S JONEEBA TIME.

I DEDICATE THIS BOOK TO GOD

For all the Good and Bad.
For Everyone who has supported me and
For all of those who tried anything to see me fail.
Because in anything you send my way,
There is a lesson to be learned to help me grow stronger.

TO MY FAMILY

Ayanna, Malika, Abdoulaye, Eladji, Reina and Morel Mouflet.

Yvette Eloise and Octave Mouflet

Suzette Mouflet

ACKNOWLEDGMENTS

A Special Thanks

To my Mentors
Aimee Cesaire, Arthur Mitchell, Miriam Makeba, Geoffrey Holder.

To my Master Teachers
Ousman Seck, Josy Michalon, Jean Claude Lamorandiere, Doudou N'Diaye Rose, Boully Sankho, Cheick Niang, Tapha Cisse, Arafan, Kemoko Sano, Ahmidou Bangoura, Germaine Acogny, Gaby Gangler, Julien Jougha, Nouksar, Ray Phillips, Omar Briant, and Jacqueline Lemoine.

To the Staff, Board of Directors, Master Teachers and Volunteers who make DJONIBA DANCE & DRUM CENTRE possible.

To my Loyal and Devoted Students, who believed in me and supported me class after class, rain, snow or sunshine.

To my Beloved Students of the Children's Program, who give me so much joy and hope for tomorrow's world.

To my Drummers and Friends who have been playing the beautiful rhythms of God that make all of us so happy in class.

To Adrienne Ingrum, without your expertise, advice, sharpness and firm belief in me, this book would not have been possible.

To the Writers, Mali and Misani, who helped me put my ideas on paper in beautiful English.

To the Experts who contributed so much, Tyran Mincey, D.C., certified applied kinesiologist, and Lara Anasaze, M.S., exercise physiologist & nutritionist.

To Stacy for introducing me to Hatherleigh Press.

To the Staff of Hatherleigh for truly believing in me: Andrew, Kevin, Tracy, Peter.

To Willie Leger, Maurice Mouflet, Evelyne Kichenama, Thierry Medelice, You Diagne and Family, the Sow Family in Malika, Mamadi Kaba, Ladji Camara, Vado Diomande, Heather Lester, Krista Retto, John Dodge, Maguette Camara, Madou Dembele, Malang Bayo, Nancy and Lincoln Field, Daniella Liebling, Nancy Sloan, Eriko Ueda, Seigo Murakami and TCA Staff, Tomo Sono Tomo, Joan van Hees, Francose Prospa and many, many more whose names are not mentioned here, but who are not forgotten.

CONTENTS

FOREWORD FROM A. DJONIBA MOUFLET   XV

PART ONE
The JONEEBA! Journey

1. *What is JONEEBA?*   3
   JONEEBA as a Total Body Workout   5
   The Vision for *JONEEBA*   6
   The Call of the Drum   8

PART TWO
Everyone Can Do JONEEBA!

2. *Who Says You Ain't Got Rhythm?*   13

3. *The "Two Left Feet" Excuse!*   17

4. *Let the Rhythm Take You Higher*   21

PART THREE
Understanding the JONEEBA! Way

5. *African History and Origin of JONEEBA*   27
   The Griot   28
   Mali: The Mandingo Culture   28
   Traditional/Folkloric African Dance vs. Choreographed/Staged
      African Dance   30
   African Dance in the U.S.   33

6. *JONEEBA Environment and Principles*   35
   Student/Teacher Behavior Principles   36
   Greetings   36
   Leaving a Master/Teacher   38
   Communication Between Master Teacher and Students   39
   Master/Teacher Rewards   39
   Peaceful and Positive Environment   40

7. *Instruments Used in a JONEEBA Class*   42
   Drums: Djimbe, Doundoun, Sangbeni and Kenkeni   42
   Other African Instruments   43

8. *What To Wear: The JONEEBA Gear*   45
   Women's and Men's Attire   46
   Footwear   47

9. *Nutrition for JONEEBA*   49
   JONEEBA and Weight Loss   49
   Getting the Most Out of *JONEEBA*   51
   Protein and Muscle Tone   52
   Water and Energy   53
   Hunger Before Class   54
   Other Healthy Eating Habits   54

10. *Injury Prevention*   57

    Maintenance and Prevention   57

    Warm-up and Cool Down   58

    Avoiding Injuries   58

PART FOUR

JONEEBA Time!

11. *The Warm-Up*   63

    Stretching   64

    Breathing   65

    Finding Your Center   66

12. *The Exercises*   67

    Start-up   67

    Floor Sequence   82

    Isolations   109

    Jumps   117

13. *The JONEEBA! Dances*   121

    Tips on How to Learn the Steps   121

    Soukous   126

    Sounou   130

    Koukou   141

    Dounoumba   149

    Manjiani   167

14. *Ending the Class*   173

    The Circle   173

    How to Join the Circle   176

    Cooling Down   176

Contents

JONEEBA! CERTIFICATIONS   177

ABOUT THE AUTHOR   179

GLOSSARY OF JONEEBA TERMS   183

GLOSSARY OF NAMES AND PLACES   185

SELECTED BIBLIOGRAPHY   187

FOREWORD

FROM A. DJONIBA MOUFLET

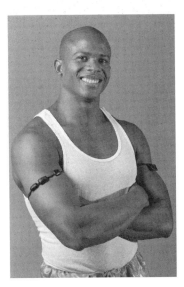

R hythm. I've always heard the rhythm. I was born with it. So were you! Listen, even as I snuggled in the dark, comforting cocoon of my mother's womb, I heard it all around me. Distinct rhythms. The rhythm of her heartbeat was just one of the rhythms which my tiny fingers would drum to during those first nine months of my life. Sometimes it would be slow and gentle, then suddenly change to fluttering, joyful beats. Throbbing. Then slow to a sensuous, passionate rhythm, only to change again to a loud, wild, fearful, racing beat, then back to a slow, calming rhythm. The heartbeat. This was the first drum beat I heard as I made my entrance into the world. My umbilical cord was cut, but my rhythm cord was, thank God, untouched. This cord remained connected to my spirit. I was given the gift of rhythm and how I chose to use that gift was up to me.

But what would I do with this gift of rhythm?

Destiny had already chartered the course, and all I had to do was follow that still small voice within to bring my gift to the world. This was my purpose for existence . . . to share my rhythm with the world.

So, my journey began. It was no coincidence that I was exposed to the drums at an early age in Martinique, and later in my teenage years when I traveled and lived in West Africa. It was here that I came to understand the connection of rhythm to the body, mind and spirit. You see, in African culture, rhythm is a natural part of life. It is celebrated by both adult and child, every second of the day, in every aspect of life at home, at school, in the workplace. I was fascinated at how the African mother at home would sing a lullaby to her infant and accentuate the melody by clapping her hands. The infant, in turn, whose spirit the rhythm had connected with, would try to clap its tiny hands, while laughing gleefully. What I realized was that the infant's body, mind and spirit were connecting. They were in harmony, which resulted in joy and peace. Over and over again, I witnessed this same phenomenon throughout the African villages. I would see women gather around a large mortar and pound cassava (tropical plants with fleshy edible rootstocks that yield a nutritious starch) or yam, with tall pestles, to a steady, rhythmic beat, while they sang. Nearby, children would play games, accompanied by a few of the young boys who would pound out a rhythm on some old log with a stick. Everyone was in unison with their bodies and minds as well as with their spirits.

The rhythm had created this union of body, mind and spirit. As I incorporated this into my lifestyle, I felt a freedom I had never felt before. I felt a oneness of mind, body and spirit and in harmony with the universe.

It was such a wonderful and empowering feeling that I had to share this experience with others. Rhythm and dance has always come natural for me. In Africa, I loved to dance in clubs and every time, before I knew it, a small crowd of people would form around me and cheer. As a matter of fact, that's how I met the highly acclaimed international performing artist, Miriam Makeba. I was dancing at the Zambezi Club (which I later found out she owned) in Guinea and everyone had stopped dancing and had formed a circle to watch me dance. Ms. Makeba and her husband were very impressed with my dancing. Realizing that I was a student studying in Guinea, they invited me to be a guest at their home. Wow! What generosity!

Mazie, (which is what those of us who were her adopted children called her) not only opened up her home to me, but she also shared the invaluable wealth of information she had garnered over the years as an international performing artist. That is what dance and rhythm has often brought to me and my life.

While living in Africa, I would go to Paris every summer to work and make money to finance my stay and tuition in Africa. Then the path took me to New York, where I attended the renowned Dance Theatre of Harlem through a scholarship and the graciousness of one of my mentors, Mr. Arthur Mitchell, whom I had met in Paris.

With many struggling moments, while still studying ballet at the Dance Theatre of Harlem, I started teaching at several dance schools. That is when I started to incorporate all that I had learned in Africa, in New York, in Martinique (yes, even when I was in my mother's womb), to develop my teaching technique. This later resulted in the creation of JONEEBA. I opened the Djoniba Dance and Drum Centre in New York City in 1994.

JONEEBA is one of the most exciting ways to work out in our time. It is a combination of three elements: my uniquely designed body stretching, strengthening, and toning warm-up; powerful West African dances done Djoniba Mouflet-style to the stimulating rhythm of the drums; and my methodical way of breaking down steps so that every person, including those who have never danced in their lives, can learn, sweat and have fun.

JONEEBA is an all-inclusive fitness program. With the JONEEBA technique, body, mind and spirit fuse. This union creates the harmony and freedom to feel and move freely with the rhythm to express yourself without inhibition, being the best you can be without competing with someone else.

This results in a powerful workout that releases all stress and allows both the inner and outer body to share equal benefits.

I have shared JONEEBA with thousands of students and visitors to my classes, including such celebrities as super-model

Roshumba, actresses Brooke Shields and Julia Roberts, the children of T.V. talk show host extraordinaire Montel Williams, and many more. Now, I would like to share my gift of rhythm with you.

It's all here in this book: *JONEEBA! The Exciting Workout and Fitness Program with the Dances and Drums of Africa.* In Part 1, you'll journey with me to West Africa, where my experiences gave me the vision and prepared me for the development and creation of the JONEEBA technique. The journey, which is both physical and spiritual, will take us to Mali, Senegal and Guinea, where I was a guest of the late President Ahmed Sekou Toure. On this journey, you will also meet some of my teachers and masters who are among the most accomplished dancers and drummers in the world. You will see how I got the "call of the drum," which you too may have but not yet know.

In Part 2 of this book, I'll share with you information about history, drums, attire, nutrition and injury prevention knowledge that is useful not only for JONEEBA, but for your entire life.

And what of Part 3? Well, it's about you, you and you! In this section, I will show you how you have everything that it takes to start JONEEBA and I will motivate you to listen. To listen? Yes! I want to teach you how to listen. That is one of the secrets of the JONEEBA technique. By learning to listen, you will be able to tap into your spirit, which then will enable you to tap into the rhythm lying dormant within you. Once you've discovered how to listen to that rhythm, then you will be able to move your body to it, and then you will transcend time and cross over into JONEEBA time. Don't worry, you'll get it.

In Part 4, it's JONEEBA time. Yes, now that you understand how it all works in your head, it's time to do it! Grab your gear, water, the JONEEBA video and CD and get busy. I will take you through the JONEEBA class in a concise, easy, fun, step-by-step method, showing you how to define and strengthen your body while getting in touch with your spirit. Your mind is already there, since you're reading this book. I will work with you, instructing you as if you were actually taking my JONEEBA class at the Djoniba Dance and Drum Centre—one of the largest multi-ethnic dance and drum centers in the world.

Touch this book. Go ahead, touch it. It's magic. You see, you are about to start on one of the most exciting journey's of your life: this fitness program! And I will be there with you, every step of the way, motivating and encouraging you, while making it an incredibly fun journey.

I guarantee JONEEBA will be a part of your lifestyle in this new millennium. Hear the rhythm. Now let the drums free your mind. Follow the spirit. It's JONEEBA time!

Have fun!
Love, Joy and Peace,
A. Djoniba Mouflet

PART 1
THE JONEEBA! JOURNEY

CHAPTER 1

WHAT IS JONEEBA?

Joneeba is not some type of "afrobics" or a mixture of some African dance steps with exercise. Why the *Exciting Workout and Fitness Program Based on the Dances and Drums of Africa*? Because it is designed to follow all the principles of exercise physiology for a complete body workout. The warm up is based on scientifically sound principles of strengthening and stretching. And the high-intensity dance from West Africa is based on scientifically sound principles of cardiovascular training. The West African dance and drum rhythm connects you to your body and soul, introducing you to a whole new level of physicality and spirituality.

JONEEBA is one of the most exciting ways to workout in the new millennium. It is a combination of three elements: my uniquely designed body stretching, strengthening, and toning warm-up; powerful West African dances done Djoniba Mouflet-style to the stimulating rhythm of the drums; and my methodical way of breaking down steps so that every person, including those who have never danced in their lives, can learn, sweat and have fun. JONEEBA is what the spirit of African dance and drumming is about—individuality, freedom of expression. That spirit that allows all to dance with their own accentuation, flavor and soul.

It's a technique that is high-energy and fun yet easy to follow, that incorporates breathing, exercises, stretches, balancing, high-impact aerobics, dance, meditation and fantastic drum music. JONEEBA is an all-inclusive fitness program that fuses style and spirit.

From a physical perspective, this technique is a whole–body workout—strengthening, toning and stretching all the muscle groups while conditioning the heart. By focusing on several groups of muscles, there is less wear and tear on any one area of the body. Instead, all the muscles get a thorough workout, which results in a strong, toned, well-defined body.

As a balance to the physical part of the workout, there is also the spiritual component of JONEEBA. The hypnotic power of JONEEBA is the drum and the rhythm, which is the foundation and core of the movements. It excites, prods, lulls, captivates, pulls, envelops and inspires you to continue on. This is where the mystical part of the JONEEBA journey begins to unfold. The ancient rhythm of the drums merges with the rhythm of your spirit, making you move with a freedom that you've never experienced before. This is the magic of JONEEBA.

The JONEEBA technique is a journey . . . your personal journey. It is a journey for your body, mind and spirit. There are no outside forces to compete with, even if you are doing your workout with a group. It is a personal journey that will awaken the world of the spirit within you. It is in this realm that the spirit, mind and body connect and there is true harmony and fulfillment.

Suddenly, you're experiencing a freedom you've never felt before. You're moving your body with a total abandonment that is truly out of this world. You are really celebrating peace and freedom. The result is that your individuality, your freedom of expression, your own accentuation and flavor are brought out as you move and begin to dance.

If you are doing your workout with a group, each student will not only experience an individual journey, but also a collective one as each spirit in the group joins together to unite with the spirit of the drum. This is an experience that has brought some of my students to such dizzying heights that they've cried out in joy.

You also get another kind of freedom with the JONEEBA technique, because it will fit into your busy lifestyle. Since the workout is inclusive, you will achieve success in less time, working on the various parts of your body together.

With the JONEEBA technique, I guarantee that you will get the workout of your life. Not only will your body look and feel great, but your spirit will be awakened to the joy of being connected to your higher self.

JONEEBA AS A TOTAL BODY WORKOUT

It is recommended that you do JONEEBA at least three times a week for optimal benefit. JONEEBA incorporates the three essential elements for a complete body workout.

Muscular Strength and Tone: The warm-up exercises combined with the high-intensity dancing strengthen all the major muscle groups in the body. During the dancing, the many "thrusting" moves particularly strengthen the muscles important for excellent posture: the muscles between the shoulder blades, the upper and lower back muscles and the neck. Since many people sit at desks in front of computers, their shoulders may become rounded forward slightly. By strengthening the key muscles for good posture, JONEEBA counteracts this effect. Strengthening the muscles also helps to prevent osteoporosis later in life. Thus, JONEEBA helps strengthen the muscles for better function, improved posture, disease prevention and a beautiful lean body.

Flexibility: Since limber muscles are important for a healthy body, the JONEEBA warm-up includes both strengthening and stretching exercises. It is designed so that the stretching exercises come second, after some initial exercises that get the blood flowing in the body and fluid flowing in the joints. This order is important for flexibility, because scientific studies show that optimal flexibility from stretching is achieved only after the muscle is already warm.

If you stretch not only after the initial exercises in the warm-up, but also after the high-intensity workout when your muscles are even warmer, you will become even more limber. The JONEEBA workout is designed not only to make the body strong, but also flexible.

Conditioning of the Heart: The high-intensity nature of JONEEBA is great for weight loss (see Ch. 9). It works in concert with the muscle toning. As you lose weight and tone the muscles, you will start to notice muscle definition throughout your body.

The high-intensity dance also conditions the heart for everyday life. After taking JONEEBA classes regularly, if you have to run a couple of blocks because you are late for the bus, for example, you not only will run faster, but also become less winded! Other cardiovascular benefits include lower cholesterol, lower blood pressure and decreased symptoms of such conditions as asthma. Clearly, JONEEBA provides muscle strength and flexibility as well as a stronger heart—a total body workout!

Remember, before embarking on this total body workout, it is recommended that you get the consent of your physician.

THE VISION FOR JONEEBA

The vision for JONEEBA came from my years of dancing and drumming. It arose from the desire to share the beauty and power of African dance and drumming with my students and to give them one basic workout that was all-inclusive.

This idea was born when I was a teenager living in Senegal, Mali and Guinea, where I studied African dance and music, jazz and modern dance, ballet and theatre. It was during this phase of my life that I first saw the connection between the physical and spiritual in the everyday lifestyle of the people. On a regular basis, what would be called in American society a big block party for the entire community of Tanabere in Senegal would be organized. These traditional parties helped Senegalese connect to and celebrate their culture, alleviate tension and stress, mark special events, have a great time and socialize. These parties, where dancing and drumming are the focal point, are part of the glue of the community, helping to heal and vitalize the bodies and minds of all those present.

At these events, several drummers gather and entice the crowd to sing, dance and jump into the mix to show off their dancing skills. But it's really not all about flashy showmanship. It's about reciprocating the energy from the drums because, at the hands of skilled musicians, African drums talk. In turn, the dancing men, women and children are moved to respond to the language of the drums with their best moves. It's a spirited conversation between drummer and dancer, and the language is urgent and yet subtle.

In Africa, dance is part of both secret rituals and everyday living. It is spiritual, religious and secular. It is purely for enjoyment and yet can be full of pomp and circumstance. African dance exists on so many planes because it addresses the physical, mental and spiritual needs of the individual and the community. It changes to mark the occasion, and it has the power to change all those who answer the call of the drums. It was there that I first got addicted to the power and spirituality of African dance and drumming and that I knew I would share it with others one day.

THE CALL OF THE DRUM

The moment I arrived in Senegal, I heard the call of the drum. There was no denying it. Back in Martinique where I was born, I had been exposed to drums. I had heard the traditional rythms of Martinique, which I later discovered were quite similar to the rhythms in West Africa. As a boy, I had even played around on drums that were made from old wine barrels. They resembled congas and were played using both the hands and feet.

But later, as I walked down the streets of Dakar, I was hypnotized by the sound of the Senegalese drums. I became obsessed by the rhythm. I had come to study dance, but the lure of the drums was overpowering. There was a connection the moment I picked up my first sabar drum. It was like thunder crashing through my body. I was hooked. How could I have ever thought you could separate the drum from the dance?

At just about the same time, I fell in love with the way a musician named Tapha Cisse played the djimbe drum. He was the drummer who played for the African dance classes I took at Mudra Afrique, a performing arts school I attended. Man, when I saw him play and heard the rhythms coming from his drum, my spirit went crazy. I was delirious. I had to learn to play the djimbe drums also. Realizing that what I was experiencing was "the call of the drums," Tapha, an extremely generous man, taught me five rhythms. I recorded these rhythms on tape and every day I would go to the beach alone and practice those five musical patterns, listening to my Walkman. Somehow, and very quickly, I picked up the rhythms, and the drum became my love. My passion. It was an uncontrollable desire that continues to this day every time I see a drum.

Watching people like my teacher, master sabar drummer Doudou N'Diaye Rose, his son Arona and Tapha Cisse play so effortlessly touched my spirit. I was determined to become a drummer. But when I played for long periods of time, my hands would throb with pain. I soon started to get big calluses which would crack as I played, or the skin of my fingers would split and blood would trickle down on top of the skins of the drum. To me, seeing the blood from my skin on the skin of the drums was profound. It was like a secret pact sealed in blood. The call of the drums had demanded a sacrificial offering from me, and I freely gave it.

I guess it was then that I knew the power of the call of the drum. It had the magic to overpower physical limitations . . . to transcend beyond pain and blood, allowing me to continue playing for long stretches of time. It seemed as if I had literally left my body behind and had soared to another realm—one of immense euphoria.

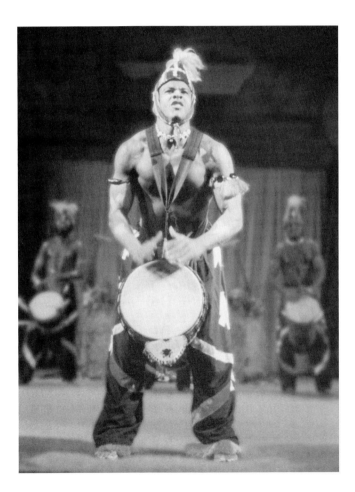

To play the drums, I realized that my body, spirit and mind had to connect. My mind commanded my hands to function and play and yet the determination could only be obtained through the spirit. Each time I played, my respect for the drums grew. Soon I realized that if I was going to play the drum well, I had to learn everything about this ancient instrument. In order to understand its magic, I had to learn its history. That's when I learned this secret of the masters. To understand the drum, I had to understand its rhythm. To understand its rhythm, I had to learn how to become one with it. But how could I do that? That's when I was taught this secret: I had to learn to listen. Not just listen with human ears, but also with spiritual ears. And so began my classes on really listening. I would do nothing but observe the master drummer play and I would do nothing but listen as the drum spoke to me. Then later I would try to replicate that same sound by first either singing or clapping the rhythmic phrasing, then replicating it on the drums. What I discovered was that once I began to incorporate the rhythms mentally, the rhythms in turn started to manifest physically. Soon, I was able to play any particular musical pattern. I was able to anticipate and hear the various breaks and know what each musical signal meant, such as when it was time to change the rhythm.

I have since gone on to become a professional drummer, and have taught many students who are now excellent djimbe drummers.

Can you hear the rhythm? If you listen closely, you too may hear the call of the drum.

PART II
EVERYONE CAN DO JONEEBA!

CHAPTER 2

WHO SAYS YOU AIN'T
GOT RHYTHM?

Rhythm is a birthright that we all share. From the moment we are con-
ceived and spend nine months growing in the protection of our
mothers' wombs, we have rhythm. It is rhythm in its most primal
form: the heartbeat.

Rhythm is a natural part of our existence in our mothers' bellies. Because
the drum of the heart is constant, we learn to move to this rhythm at the ear-
liest stages of being. From the time our mothers wake up and eat a meal to going to work to finally going to sleep, we have this rhythm. Its pulse is always
surrounding us, rocking us, nurturing our tiny spirits. After birth, our natural
rhythms will either be cultivated or seemingly disappear.

In African culture, rhythm is organic. It is celebrated everywhere and nur-
tured from the very beginning of a child's life. A mother might sing a lullaby
to her toddler and accentuate the melody by clapping her hands.

Women in some villages will gather around a large mortar and pound cassava or yam with tall pestles to a steady beat while they sing songs to make the
work go by a little faster.

Their children will be nearby, playing games as their mothers work. Young boys learn musical games early on and might gather around an old log and pound it with sticks to create their own music. When a group of drummers get together, adults and children often form a spontaneous circle around them and take turns jumping into the center to dance.

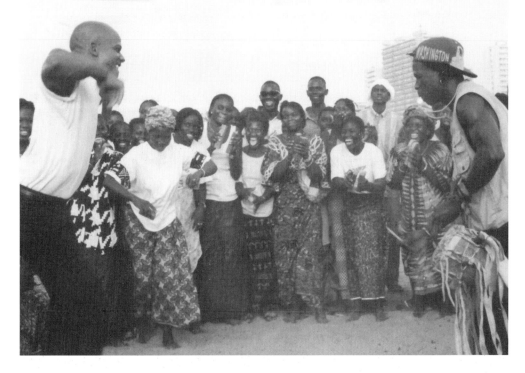

Special occasions like weddings or parties aren't the only places to celebrate rhythm there. Clapping, singing, dancing and the playing of musical instruments are all a part of the continent's cultural history and happen naturally on a regular basis. African people from the Caribbean and North and South American countries stayed grounded in their original African rhythm, despite separation from their Motherland. From samba to salsa to jazz to zouk or the blues, rhythm has remained engraved in our souls. Which brings us to the question, Do people who are not of African descent have rhythm? To this, I say, again: Everyone is born with rhythm. Different groups of people, however, have developed their rhythm more than others.

One of the things which I incorporate into JONEEBA is teaching people to hear. Yes, hear. Really hear the music. Only when you are able to hear the music will you be able to move freely. How does one hear? It is by listening. Really listening. Listening to the rhythm is the core of the success of JONEEBA. My students become so tuned in and turned on to listening to the rhythms of the drums that the mind-body-spirit connection is made quickly and they're able to dance freely, with rhythm, to the rhythm of the drums.

One of my students, who has been attending my classes for a year, told me: "I always had rhythm—for a white a girl!" That is, until she took a JONEEBA class and the drummers started to play. She could dance to the beat, she said, but when the drummers played the break (a musical phrase that signals change) she was clueless. A big issue for her was the changes in the rhythm, which are much more intricate in African drumming than in popular dance music. She would have been doing the same step for the whole class if I hadn't helped her to really listen to the breaks. What helped her the most was when I had the students sing and clap the change in the beat, so she could hear it in the music. Those of you who are doing JONEEBA at home, this is exactly what you will hear on my CD, "JONEEBA Drums for Your Soul."

Another student, an Asian woman who has been attending my class for the past five years, told me she loved coming to move and dance to the African drums, but that she sometimes felt awkward doing the steps and hearing the rhythms. She further confided that she was a "very slow learner." I suggested that she start taking my djimbe drum class to get a better understanding of the music, which would also help her feel the dances more. She later told me that taking the djimbe classes changed everything for her. She could finally hear the rhythm and the breaks. She understood the relationship

If you can walk, you can dance.

between when her feet should start moving, the transition from the break to the rhythm, and when to move. She was amazed. She could not get all of that before she started doing it with her hands.

Trust me. We all have rhythm. Some of us just need to work on listening to it. Here are a few suggestions to help you to tap into your rhythmic inner self:

- **Listening:** Focus on the structure of the dance's rhythms. Listen for the musical phrasing. Identify the breaks.

- **Clapping:** Observe the various patterns being played. Try to clap out the breaks.

- **Singing:** Vocalize the rhythms. Sing the doundoun, or bass drum, pattern. Sing the djimbe's main rhythm. Sing the breaks.

- **Listen to the CD:** "JONEEBA Drums for Your Soul," which takes you through the rhythms and breaks for various dances.

And remember, everyone has rhythm. Some just need to develop it, that's all. And you can with JONEEBA. I will take you through a step-by-step method to help you understand.

CHAPTER 3

THE "TWO LEFT FEET" EXCUSE!

When Ousman Seck, my first African dance teacher, danced, he was poetry in motion. His feet would hit the floor quickly and deliberately, mapping out the dance's pattern. His strong legs and upper body moved with energetic force and grace. His long arms captured time and space. His head helped punctuate the movements.

I remember that when I saw Ousman dance, my spirit reassured me I could follow him. Something deep within seemed to remember the movements and so it came naturally to me.

Dance has always come naturally to me. I remember back in Martinique some of my fellow students would struggle to get the steps, and I would catch on really fast. Now I realize they were fighting with their spirits instead of letting their spirits work through them.

Hundreds of excited students come through the doors of the Djoniba Dance and Drum Centre for JONEEBA classes. My initial advice to each one is to forget about everyone else in the class except the teacher, the drummer, the drums and yourself. You're in this JONEEBA class to dance and you will dance and move like you've never done before. And then the questions start. "Will I be on the beat?" "Isn't there some kind of musical cue to let you know when to change the dance step?" "What are the dance steps anyway?" "What was the name of this dance again?" All sorts of questions. You may not learn everything at first, but with your patience and my methodical teaching, you will learn in time. Over the years, my technique has helped turn many people who thought they had two left feet into good dancers.

A student once told me that my class is one of the few where she felt she could really learn as a beginner. She said she was able to grasp it because of the way I broke down the steps. In my class, most beginners get it. Yet, the class never stops. I make it fun so that you don't realize how hard you're working until your JONEEBA wear is soaking wet. Since I give my all and I love what I am doing, my students can't help but go full out and love it too.

Another student who has been taking my class since 1990 said he had always wanted to dance, but when he started taking my JONEEBA class, he was a perfect example of what he called two left feet. "When everybody went right, I went left. It was so bad

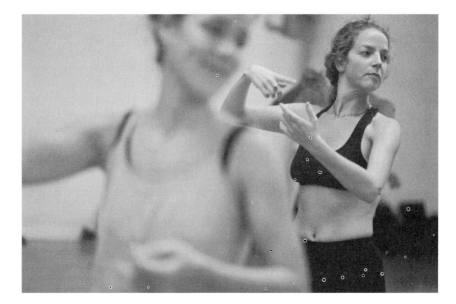

that people would laugh at me," he now says. I remember telling this student not to worry, that I would make him a dancer. He did turn into a good dancer—so much so, that he's now performing all over the country.

For those of you who may get a little shy when the drums start to play, here are a few tips to help you loosen up and get on the right foot.

> ∽ **Be Patient:** An African proverb says you can only eat the elephant one bite at a time. That means take your time and really give yourself a chance to learn the moves in JONEEBA. You can't expect to be able to dance Manjiani (see description in Part 4, Chapter 13) perfectly if you just learned it. Be patient with yourself.

Remember, getting the dance moves down in JONEEBA requires an adjustment period. I'm here to steer you through. I'll break down all the steps so that you can pick them up in a way you'll understand. In time and with my guidance, you'll get the moves.

> ∽ **Set Goals:** Give yourself a set period of time to learn JONEEBA. Lower the bar of expectations—now that you're learning to be patient with yourself—and decide that within, say, six months you will have learned many of the JONEEBA moves.

Remember, practice makes perfect. The more classes you take, or the more you practice at home and watch the video and play the tapes, the better you'll get!

> ∽ **Don't Compete and Don't Compare:** Everyone is different. We learn things at different paces, and we all have different ways of learning.

You can only eat the elephant one bite at a time.

The "Two Left Feet" Excuse!

Some people come to class and get all the steps the same day. They can pick up all the steps that I show them without much effort. Some happen to be coordinated dancers and athletes, others have learned to tap into their spirit to listen to their rhythm telling them how to move to the rhythm of the drum. But the majority of my students need to be patiently guided through every step.

One young woman recently took her first class with me. She had come with a girlfriend and had a background in Indian dance. She knew that she had rhythm and that she could dance. But JONEEBA was different.

"I'm feeling the rhythm. But sometimes I'm looking at others to try to figure out the step," she told me. Then she admitted that she wanted to be cool like my more advanced students, who were getting the steps faster.

My advice to her was not to be like anybody but herself, which is also my advice to you. That is the beauty of JONEEBA. It allows you to express your individuality. So be unique. Remember, there's no one else quite like you.

⌒ *Have Fun:* A workout should be enjoyable, not drudgery.

Remember, JONEEBA is fun. It's spirited and, yes, it's challenging. You're not auditioning. You're doing it because you love the way it makes you feel as you get in shape. So lighten up, hear the rhythm. Follow your spirit.

JONEEBA!

CHAPTER 4

LET THE RHYTHM
TAKE YOU HIGHER

The power of JONEEBA is the drum. It is the foundation and core of the movements. It excites, prods, lulls, captivates, pulls, envelops and inspires you to continue on. It gives you the freedom to open yourself up to the rhythm. Once you find that rhythm and give in to its mighty force, your body and your mind transcend to the next level: body meeting spirit. The rhythm of the drums allows you to abandon your inhibitions and transcend unto the highest level—the spirit. The dance and drumming have a hypnotic power that makes you forget everything but the rhythm. It allows you to release stress, and at the same time, it puts you totally in balance physically, mentally and spiritually. It's almost like going back into the womb. Back then, in that perfect place, you moved to the rhythm of your mother's heartbeat. That was your pulse, your inner guide. It was your compass and your balance. Now, you're moving to the rhythm of your own spirit. The rhythm in JONEEBA allows you to go back to that place of innocence and perfection, while at the same time dealing with your higher self.

In JONEEBA, I teach West African dance movement. The drums tell you when to begin dancing. A "break" (the musical phrase that signals a change) tells you when to stop. Eventually, you will hear and learn those different breaks and rhythms. In the djimbe orchestra (the djimbe, doundoun, songba, and kenkeni drums), the drums guide your movements. They call you to dance, and their rhythms and accentuation help you to understand the movements.

Once the drummers begin to play, the energy level escalates and the dancers are buoyed by their rhythms. They are spurred on by the drums, which keep their energy levels high. The drums speak to you

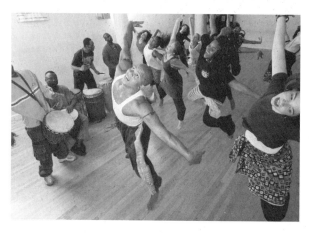

with passion and you must respond the same way . . . with passion. And you want to! The drums make you want to give it up, work your body until you're completely cleansed and need to go somewhere and just sit down. But you can't because the drums won't let you.

With JONEEBA, it's hard to get bored because the drums inspire you to move your body. And that's important in any fitness program—to find that something that keeps you going, inspires you to continue.

The sound waves of the drum are very powerful. In both traditional and pop African music, you can hear the drum's call. When I teach my classes, I use live drummers. If you're doing JONEEBA at home, a drumming CD will do just as well. During the warm-up, I sometimes use modern band music from Africa and the Caribbean. I include soukous from Congo, m'balax from Senegal, and zouk from Martinique. I like to mix it up because it represents all of the musical styles I love that are now categorized as World Music. Record labels like Mango, Putumayo and Island Records have been introducing U.S. audiences to African pop music for years. African singers and musicians like Youssou N'Dour and Thione Seck of Senegal, Salif Keita of Mali, King Sunny Ade of Nigeria, Angelique Kidjo of Benin, and Tabu Ley Rochereau of Congo have found their way

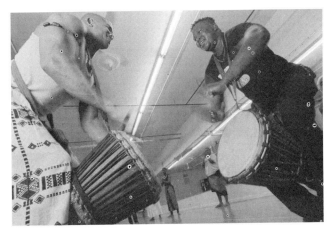

onto U.S. music charts and into personal CD collections.

When a group of skilled musicians plays the drums, the music can be mesmerizing. In my classes, I usually have several musicians/drummers from West Africa, the United States, and the Caribbean playing together; among them are some of the hottest around today. They include my lead drummers Madou Dembele and Fode Bangoura, as well as Fode Cissoko, Maguette Camara, Vado Diomande, Joe Barnes, Atito Gohi, Moko Camara, Lansana Toure and Mangay Silla. The musical accompaniment for the dance is a huge draw for my students, as it will be for those of you who listen to the CD at home.

When listening to talented drummers such as Madou Dembele, Ladji Camara, Mamady Keita, Doudou N'Diaye Rose, Cheick Tairoumbaye or Gregory Ince, to name a few, a shift in energy happens. Their music takes you to a trance-like state that can make you and everybody around

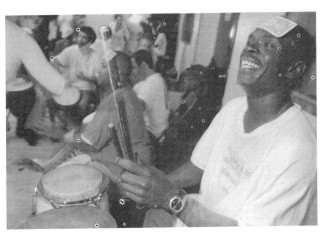

you scream. Then you know you're in the presence of a master drummer or a "djimbefola." According to Ladji Camara, one of the first members of Les Ballets Africains de Keita Fodeba, the term "djimbefola" used to be a derogatory term for a djimbe player. Over the years, it has changed completely to describe a djimbe master as someone who knows the secrets of the djimbe's language. The secrets are passed from masters to students. It is only by practicing for many years that you can make the djimbe talk, sing and move your spirit.

Move to the rhythm of your own spirit

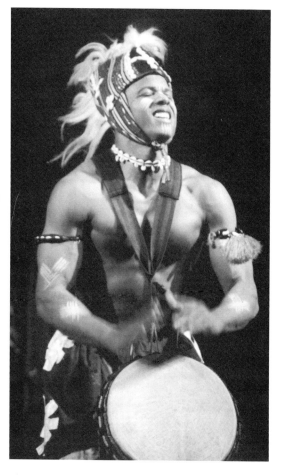

When I play the djimbe, it lifts me spiritually, mentally and physically to new heights. As the years go by, it gets even stronger and has me feeling as though I am in a trance. That is what other djimbefolas say also, whether they are born in Brooklyn, Martinique, or Africa.

If you listen closely to the sound of the drum when you dance, it is sure to elicit in you the same joy, freedom and happiness. And in turn, you will undoubtedly dance much better. So let the rhythms take you higher and let your spirit dance!

PART III:
UNDERSTANDING
THE
JONEEBA WAY

CHAPTER 5

AFRICAN HISTORY AND ORIGIN OF JONEEBA

To understand JONEEBA, we need to understand the origins of the dances and the history of the people from which they came, but we also need to understand the differences between staged and traditional/folkloric African dance.

Living in West Africa for many years, I got to learn the dance and drum, and most importantly, the culture and the way of life. My research also involved interviews and audio and video recording. I traveled to villages and cities in Guinea, Mali and Senegal, and I was fortunate to have griot men and women (see next section) who were open to me about the culture. I also was acquainted with some West African scholars and anthropologists whose books I read or who shared their knowledge with me.

Djibril Tamsir Niane, a respected historian and anthropologist from Senegal, explains in his book *Research on the Mali Empire in the Middle Ages* that most of the anthropologists and historians who studied that period based their research on writings from Arabs and Muslims as well as books and notes from French and Portuguese traders. But a big part of their research also came from the griot.

THE GRIOT

Some historians have disregarded the importance of the griot as a keeper of the culture because they maintain an oral history. Historically, griots always have been the transmitters of the history of the people. They are basically walking libraries. They are singers and talkers who herald the history of the culture. They have a real method of keeping this tradition and have passed it on from family to family, from father to son.

For important occasions, such as weddings, births, passages of power and death, the griot sings and pontificates about the history of the king, the town and its heroes. In addition to the singing griots, there are also griots who play the drums and other instruments. They are still part of the culture today.

THE MALI EMPIRE

The African dance and drum music that I teach in JONEEBA has its roots in the culture of the Manding, who are also called Mandingo, Mandinka, Malinke or Djoula (tradesman). The Manding trace their roots back to the old Mali Empire. The Mali Empire, which rose to power under Sundiata Keita in 1235 AD, was one of the largest and most powerful in Africa. According to historians, the Manding settled along the Gambia and Casamance Rivers in the 13th century. As the empire grew, it included parts of present-day Mali, Niger, Burkina Faso, Guinea, Guinea-Bissau, Mauritania, Senegal and all of Gambia.

At the Berlin Conference in 1885, the European countries of France, England, Germany and Portugal divided Africa into countries among themselves, with little regard for traditional cultural, ethnic and tribal boundaries.

The country called Mali became a conglomerate of Malinke (also known as Bambara), Peul and other ethnic groups. Guinea was made up of Malinke, Susu, Peul, Baga and others. This same

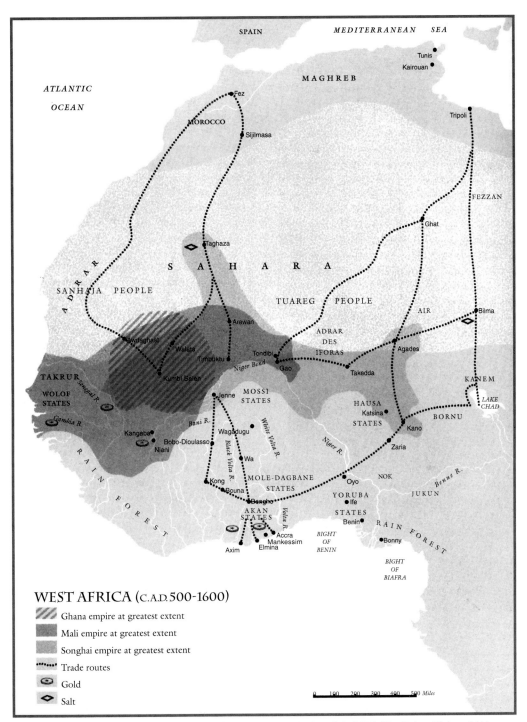

WEST AFRICA (C.A.D. 500-1600)

- ///// Ghana empire at greatest extent
- ▓▓▓ Mali empire at greatest extent
- ░░░ Songhai empire at greatest extent
- ••••• Trade routes
- ◉ Gold
- ◆ Salt

0   100   200   300   400   500 *Miles*

Source: Reprinted with permission by The McGraw-Hill Companies in Boahen, A.A. (1971). *The Horizon History of Africa.*
New York: American Heritage Publishing.

pattern occurred in Senegal and the Ivory Coast. What resulted was that the Mandingo culture was spread into these different countries. Although the fundamental principles of the cultural arts remained the same, the separation created differences within the once common dance and music cultures. The dounoumba dance and music, for example, was and continues to this day to be executed differently in Senegal, Mali and Guinea, although its foundation is rooted in the Mandingo culture. Because of this cultural diffusion, it is incorrect to claim that one version of dounoumba is more authentic or original than another.

TRADITIONAL FOLKLORIC AFRICAN DANCE vs. STAGED / CHOREOGRAPHED AFRICAN DANCE

In the 1950s, traditional folkloric dance and music, which had been performed in villages for celebrations, religious and ritual occasions, were taken out of their authentic settings to be choreographed for the stage. The godfather of staged African dancing is Keita Fodeba, who founded Les Ballets Africains de Keita Fodeba in Paris in 1952. At the time, Fodeba was a young Guinean scholar who aspired to present traditional African music and dance in Western venues. He modeled his staging and choreography after European standards for staged shows. From 1952 to 1958, his company performed throughout the world.

When Guinea gained independence from France on Oct. 2, 1958, Sekou Toure, the new president of the Guinea Republic, invited Fodeba back home with his company to create a national ballet. In the 1960s, a number of performers from various ethnic groups and villages were selected and Les Ballets Africains de Guinea was formed. Now, under one cultural umbrella, all of Guinea's different ethnic groups were exposed firsthand to each others' cultures. Malinkes would sing in Susu, Peuls would dance Malinke dances, and Susus would play Malinke rhythms.

Under Fodeba's adept direction and his lofty vision, this elite company dazzled. Sweeping, clean lines. Powerful, wild movements. Graceful, intricate choreography. Lavish, colorful costumes. Les Ballet Africains set the standard for professional African ballet.

Its success spurred the creation of other professional African dance troupes across the continent, many of whom modeled their companies after the prestigious Les Ballets Africains.

Fodeba's new standard and vision of staged African dance brought him great success but also much criticism. In 1959, Leopold Sedar Senghor, the first president of Senegal and a noted writer and scholar, applauded Les Ballet Africains de Keita Fodeba in his book, *Liberte, Negritudé et Humanisme.*

"The evening of June 28, 1959, that I spent watching the ballet of Keita Fodeba in the national theatre of the palace of Dakar was exceptional....But I was reading critiques saying this of Mr. Fodeba: 'Fodeba Keita has betrayed black Africa. He's far from representing those dances that are done in the villages in the moonlight around fire.' Dear Sir, I answered to myself, you've mistaken folklore and art. The village is not a stage. The theatre is another space and another time. It is not a question to reproduce exactly, to photograph popular dances. It is a question to create new works inspired by the popular dances but at the same time keeping the spirit. That is what Keita Fodeba has done."[1]

Clearly, folkloric African dance in the village is very different from choreographed African dance for the stage, and President Senghor understood this.

Interestingly, the same issues of authenticity in traditional African dance vs. staged/choreographed African dance discussed by Senghor in 1959 still exist today. Many people in the West, lacking information about the history and the culture, have mistaken authentic African dance and music from the forests or the villages with African dance choreographed for the stage.

In the Western world today, what we see on stage and learn in class is mostly African dance and music that has been modified, choreographed and composed in national and local companies of African cities. Most of the teachers and musicians who now live in the Western world, including myself, are teaching dances learned from those West African companies, and from master/genius choreographers such as Kemoko Sano of the National Ballet of Guinea and Boully Sankho of the National Ballet of Senegal, who inspired the scene for traditional dance, but modified and choreographed the dance for the stage.

Most of the dances learned in class are not those done by a campfire in a grass skirt, unless you go to Africa, find a village, get initiated, and learn only three steps after all this travelling! African dance done in the villages is not choreography of many steps, but rather a simple dance of a few steps. It's like learning the original slide from your uncle compared to learning a choreographed version of the slide, with complicated steps and turns, to be performed on an MTV video. Anyone claiming authenticity is usually doing so for financial gain and to attract uninformed students or audiences.

In my discussion with former President Ahmed Sekou Toure, whom I had the honor to meet, he insisted that it is creativity that will keep African dance a powerful art form. That is why he sent many young Guineans to study acrobatics, costuming and stage decor in other countries such as Korea and encouraged the development of original steps from the village into more elaborate and refined choreography.

West African dance is now a recognized art form, just like jazz dance, yoga or karate. You don't have to be born in America to learn or teach jazz dance or hip-hop, nor in Japan to teach or learn karate, nor in Africa to teach or learn African dance and drums, but you do need the willingness to truly capture the spirit and essence of the dance and music.

AFRICAN DANCE IN THE UNITED STATES

When Fodeba's troupe traveled to the United States in the 1950s, Americans got a taste of the incredible dance and drum culture of Guinea. Their mesmerizing music, dazzling dance, and acrobatics

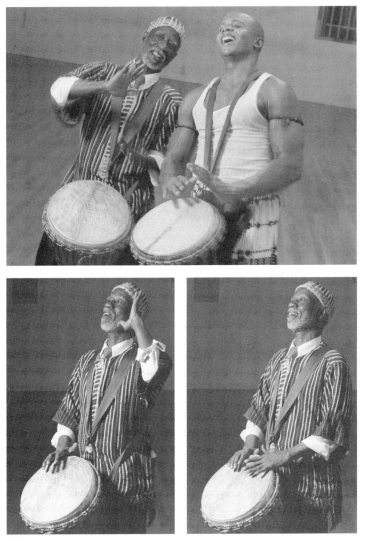

"Papa" Ladji Camara

captured the American audience, inspiring them to learn African dance and drums.

Ladji Camara, also known as "Papa Ladji," a former member of Les Ballets Africains, is said to have been the first African to introduce the djimbe to Americans. After several years of performing with the national ballet as a drummer, Camara relocated to New York City and taught numerous Americans djimbe drumming, dances, songs and African culture.

Nigerian musician Babatunde Olatunji also had come to the United States in the 1950s to pursue an education at Morehouse College, then went to New York City to further his studies. He formed the Institute for the Study of African Culture, a center dedicated to the study of African music and dance. Olatunji teamed up with Ladji Camara, who taught and performed djimbe with him.

Once Africans began to emigrate to the United States, the culture of West African dance and drumming began to take root. Americans, especially those of African descent, learned from Africans and began to create their own traditional dance and drumming ensembles.

African-Americans such as Chief Bey, Chuck Davis, Dinizulu, Katherine Dunham and Melvin Deal, to name a few, were some of the first to tap into this cultural exchange with their African heritage. Today, the list continues to grow, and schools such as the Djoniba Dance and Drum Centre serve as major institutions for the new students who want to learn African dance and culture and for those who hear the call of the drum.

CHAPTER 6

JONEEBA ENVIRONMENT AND PRINCIPLES

J ONEEBA is about freedom—the freedom to know yourself and explore your identity in a positive and supportive environment, whether it is at my dance and drum center or in a space you have created at home for your new fitness program. In the case of a class in a studio, as you dance with other students, you start to feed off of each others' energy. With time, you begin to cut your own identity in the class, putting your own flavor into each dance. Then something wonderful often starts to happen. The more you come to class, the more you begin to feel as though you are a part of something different and special—a big family. In time, you make friends with fellow dancers whom you see on a regular basis.

If you're at home, I encourage you to create this feeling of community. That's what Djoniba Dance and Drum Centre is about—people from all walks of life dancing and drumming together, bringing their different styles to JONEEBA and having a good time. This environment should be mutually supportive. As you do JONEEBA, you give support to your teacher, who passes on to you his or her lifelong knowledge. Because his or her spirit is connecting to your spirit, it is important to understand and follow certain codes and standards relating to teacher-student relationships.

Give credit and remain loyal to your teacher for the lifelong knowledge passed on to you.

STUDENT / TEACHER BEHAVIOR PRINCIPLES

In Africa, you are taught that no matter how much you pay your teacher, you can never repay him or her for the lifelong knowledge and secrets passed on to you. Even if you are not a professional dancer and drummer, learning even a few dances from a teacher requires this mentorship. Your first teacher—the one who taught you the basics—becomes your mother-master or father-master. It is imperative to give credit openly, remain loyal, protect and give gratitude and support to all of your teachers, and especially to your first teacher, regardless of whom you may study with later.

The following codes and standards, though not necessarily applicable in the same way, are excellent guidelines to help you throughout life in teacher/student relationships.

GREETINGS

JONEEBA students should greet their master teacher in a respectful manner. Women should place their hands on knees with a slight knee bow followed by any other form of greeting permitted.

The men should greet with their hands at their backs with a slight chest bow and/or with a handshake by holding the right forearm with the left hand.

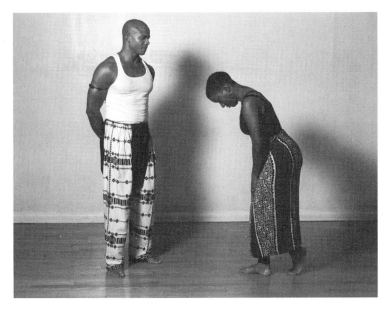

Woman's Greeting

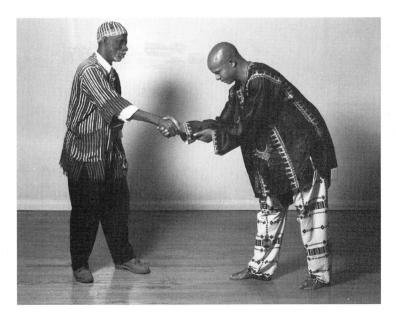

Man's Greeting

Joneeba Environment and Principle

37

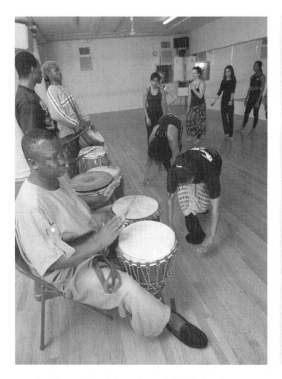

Suggestions:

(1) At the beginning of class or any point during class, greet the students next to you by introducing yourself.

(2) At the end of class, greet and thank your master teacher with the same beginning bow.

(3) Thank the spirit of the drum by touching the floor.

Students thanking the spirit of the drum.

LEAVING A MASTER TEACHER

It is important and only natural that in order to develop and grow in your discipline, a student who has studied with one master teacher will leave to start studying with other master teachers. Leaving includes not just moving to a different city, but also studying with a different teacher in the same studio or town, whether the transition is due to a change in your schedule, or a need for new knowledge, etc.

When you are ready to leave your first master teacher to take other classes, a proper transition is necessary. The separation should be done respectfully and with much gratitude.

You should inform your teacher of your intentions to study elsewhere by letter or card, thanking him or her for all that was given. This note should be accompanied by some sort of modest gift or souvenir to show your gratitude.

It is also important to inform your new teacher of your previous master teacher and his or her background. You should not study with anyone who does not respectfully understand and accept your previous training.

Even after you're no longer studying with your first master teacher, you should pay him or her a visit and take a class there once in a while.

COMMUNICATION BETWEEN MASTER TEACHER AND STUDENTS

Teachers are human and therefore imperfect, so if they do something wrong or something that may have disturbed you, speak or write to them directly and stay positive to resolve the matter. It is disrespectful to speak or complain to others about your teachers.

MASTER TEACHER REWARDS

I have had students who have studied with me for more than 10 years, who have also studied with other master teachers and have become amazing dancers. They still attend my beginner class once in a while and they stay in touch with me. Additionally, they acknowledge what was passed on to them in the JONEEBA classes they attended. One student even named her daughter after me. Even though this student is now studying with other master teachers, her daughter has attended my children's program, Djoniba Dance and Drum Kids, for seven years, since she was five years old. It's such things that make teaching JONEEBA a blessing.

Master teachers may form a dance company and give performances with students who are studying with them or who have studied with them in the past. I have had my own dance company for years, and some of its members are my dance and drum students and other master teachers. My students also get to perform at an annual Dance and Drum festival that is produced by D.D.D.C. in June in New York.

Many students have come through my classes over the years. I have given them a foundation in African dance and drumming and have taught them various dances and rhythms from West Africa, as well as giving them knowledge that they can carry anywhere they go. In my class, my students have gained confidence in themselves. This is evidenced when I see how my students have branched out all across the country, taking with them the fundamentals and movement vocabulary that will allow them to take any other dance class or fitness program.

PEACEFUL AND POSITIVE ENVIRONMENT

JONEEBA promotes all the benefits of fitness, spirituality and respect for one another. JONEEBA promotes a community of open-minded, free and down-to-earth people sharing a beautiful art form, respecting each other, and having fun together in a positive and healthy environment regardless of color, religion, or gender. Everyone should feel welcome and wanted.

If you would like to create such an environment, you can start your own JONEEBA class by becoming a certified JONEEBA instructor. (See the back of the book for more information.)

CHAPTER 7

INSTRUMENTS USED IN A JONEEBA CLASS

THE DRUMS:
DJIMBE, DOUNDOUN, SANGBENI, AND KENKENI

The most widely recognized African drum is the djimbe drum. The djimbe is carved from a piece of solid wood. A goat or cow skin then is stretched tautly over the open top and an intricate pattern of cord lacing is pulled around the bowl of the shell to control the drum's pitch. The djimbe is played widely in Africa, and it is considered an integral part of ceremonial and festive occasions.

The origin of the djimbe has been debated for a long time. Some musicians will say that the djimbe is from Guinea, while others argue that it is from Mali. Both of

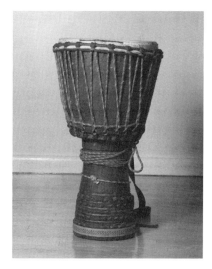

Djimbe

these theories are true because Mali and Guinea were both part of the Mali Empire before colonization. The djimbe originated during the time of the Mali Empire and was created by the Malinke people.

Within the djimbe orchestra, each drum plays a particular musical pattern. The lead djimbe player has the most freedom of expression musically, and this drum is in constant conversation with the dancers. The lead player tells dancers when to start, when to change from one step to the next, and when to stop. The lead djimbe inspires the dancers to dance. Other djimbe players stick to a regular pattern.

The doundoun, a two-headed drum made of either wood or a large metal container, is the bass and adds funk to the music. The sangbeni and kenkeni add higher bass tones. The sangbeni is a mid-size two-headed drum that has a higher pitch than the doundoun,

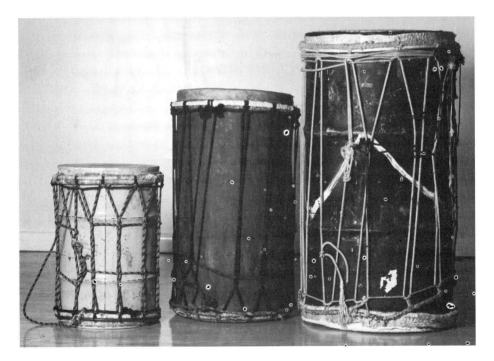

From left to right: sangbeni and two doundoun drums of different sizes
(The kenkeni, not pictured, is smaller than the sangbeni.)

JONEEBA!

which it complements. The kenkeni is the smallest of the two-headed drums and has the highest tone. Both the songba and the kenkeni often have a metal bell attached to accentuate the music. Played separately, these musical phrases are simple mono-rhythms. But when the orchestra comes together, the music becomes polyrhythmic, a soulful mix of percussion.

OTHER AFRICAN INSTRUMENTS:
THE BALAPHON, KORA, AND SHEKERE

Though the drum is the instrument most associated with Africa, in JONEEBA, we also use other musical instruments. Among them are the balaphon, which is Africa's version of the modern xylophone; the kora, a 21-string harp/lute, which is the traditional instrument used by Malinke griots, or praise singers; and the shekere, which is a large gourd rattle played in West Africa.

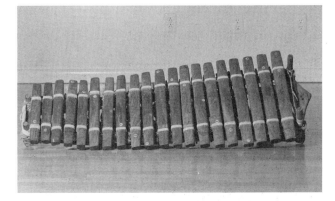

Balaphon

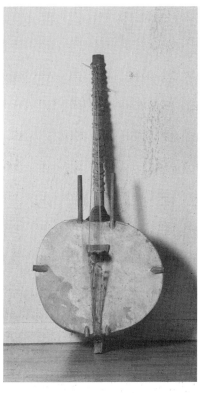

Kora

Instruments Used in a Joneeba Class

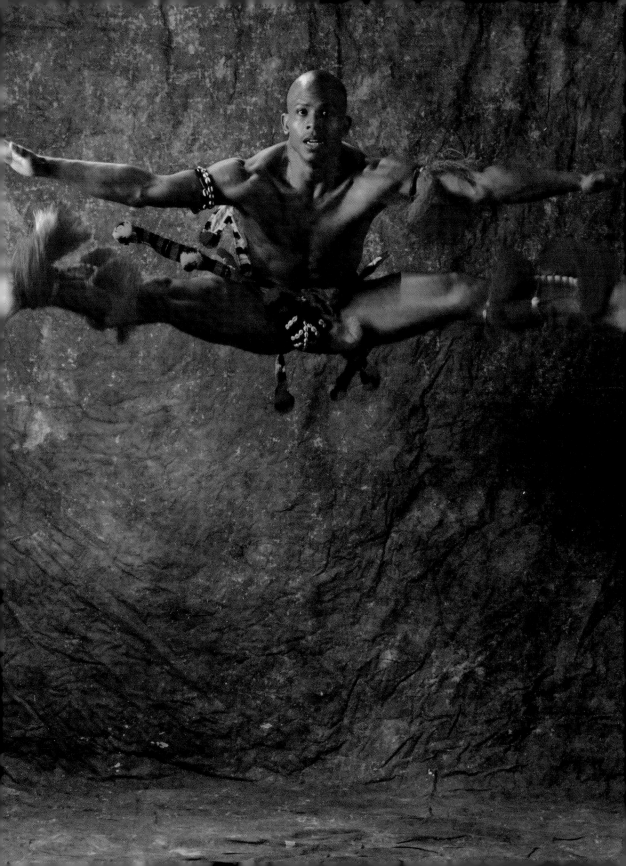

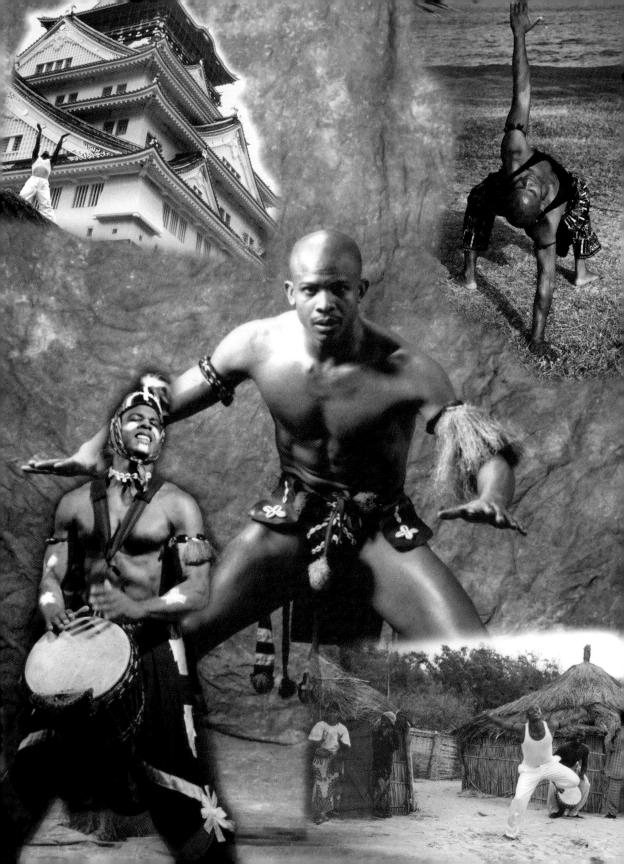

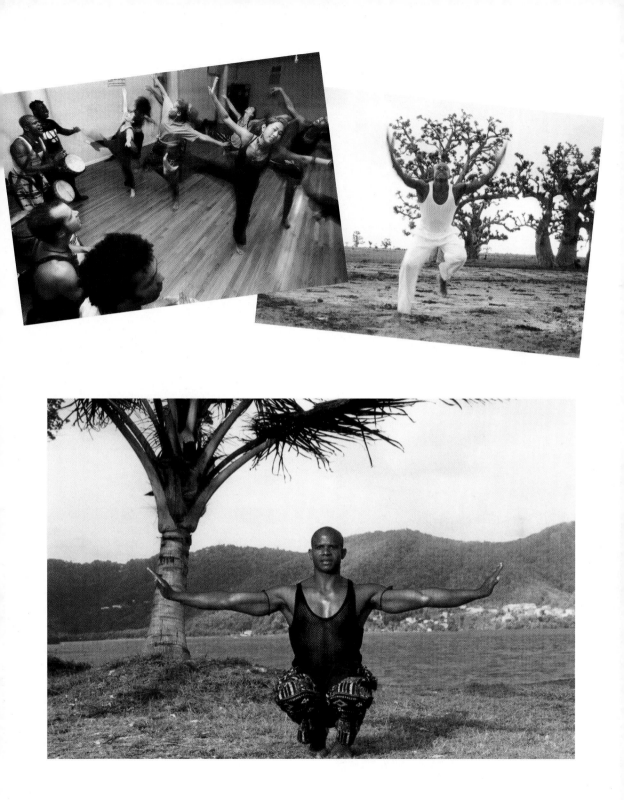

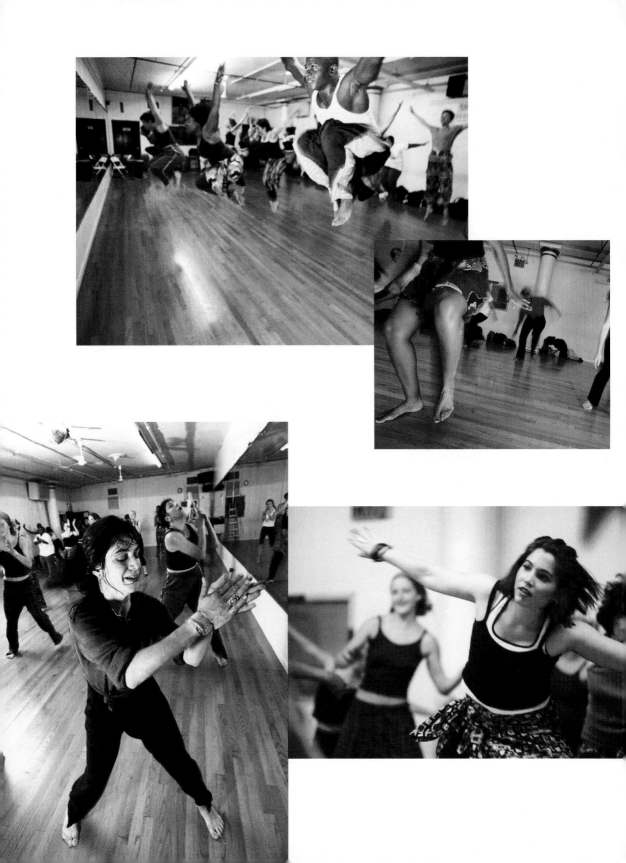

CHAPTER 8

WHAT TO WEAR?
THE JONEEBA GEAR

Workout attire can make exercising a comfortable experience or a disconcerting and even embarrassing event.

Some people may think that taking a JONEEBA class requires dressing up like the pictures you see in National Geographic magazine and anthropology books that portray Africans in the most rustic or regal settings: Wodaabe men painted in makeup making faces as they try to impress female suitors; Masai warriors slathered in ocher and wearing very little; Ashanti royalty wrapped in yards of kente cloth; or Congolese men dancing in grass skirts.

They work for *National Geographic*, but not for my class. To do JONEEBA, you should wear comfortable attire. You need to feel free as you do the movements. Some women come in sports bras and tights or leggings. Men tend to come in sweat pants and a T-shirt. Some even come in shorts. If they feel comfortable in the gym/sport look, that's fine.

I recommend, however, that as you become more confident and comfortable in the class, that you start wearing JONEEBA gear. You see, for any dance discipline there is a uniform. In ballet, although you can wear sweat pants, it feels and looks more like a ballet class the moment you put on a leo-tard, tights, and ballet slippers. Your whole attitude changes. You feel like you're a ballet dancer. The same thing happens when you wear JONEEBA gear.

WOMEN'S AND MEN'S ATTIRE

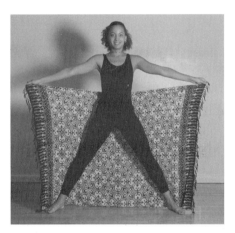

Suggested attire for a JONEEBA class is the lapa for women and the chaya or the straight pant for men.

The lapa is similar to a sarong. It is a piece of fabric, preferably African, that is wrapped around the waist and tied or tucked in the back. In Africa they are worn by women every day.

The chaya pants are loose-fitting pants that usually have a drawstring or elastic waistband. They have a

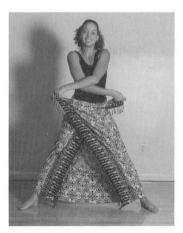
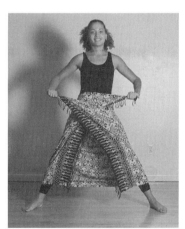
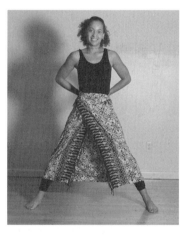

Woman tying a lapa

JONEEBA!

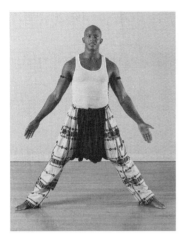

dropped crotch with draped fabric that accents this area. They are worn in Africa and the Middle East. Light straight stretch pants can also be worn.

When wearing a lapa, ladies must remember to wear shorts or tights underneath in case the lapa becomes loose. Once you start wearing JONEEBA attire, your whole attitude will suddenly change and you will start feeling like a JONEEBA dancer. You will feel closer to the culture, and it does make the class colorful and cheerful. Colors make you feel happy, so wear them to put a smile on your face.

FOOTWEAR

JONEEBA footwear is quite inexpensive. As a matter of fact, I think my workout requires the cheapest footwear around: your bare feet! It is recommended to take classes barefoot, unless you have problems with your feet, legs or back. In that case, you should consult your doctor for proper footwear.

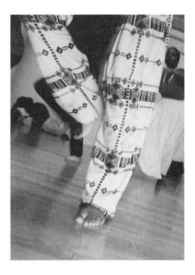

CHAPTER 9

NUTRITION FOR JONEEBA

A JONEEBA class is just one part of maintaining a healthy body. The second major component is good nutrition. The two work together. When they are balanced, most people feel and look better. I try to eat as healthily as possible without overdoing it. But whatever you choose, it must be what works for your body.

The following are some suggestions about exercise and nutrition recommended for maintaining a healthy and beautiful body. You may or may not use them, but at least you have the information to provide you with a choice.

JONEEBA AND WEIGHT LOSS

In order to understand how to maintain a lean body or lose weight, you should understand the concept of the target heart rate zone and calories.

TARGET HEART RATE

If you have cardiovascular problems, consult with your physician to make sure this type of high-intensity workout is safe for you. Only your physician can accurately calculate the heart rate (number of heart beats per minute) safe for you during exercise.

Your target heart rate zone can be determined by subtracting your age from 220, (the calculated number of the recommended exercise target heart range) and then multiplying this number by two different percentages: 60% and 75%.

We can calculate the target heart rate for a 40-year-old individual using this example:

$$220 - 40 = 180$$
$$180 \times 60\% = 108$$
$$180 \times 75\% = 135$$

The target heart rate zone for the 40-year-old individual is 108 to 135 beats per minute.

> To determine your heart rate during exercise
>
> 1. Count the number of beats using your pulse at your wrist.
>
> 2. After fifteen seconds, stop counting.
>
> 3. Multiply that number by 4.

During exercise, when your heart rate is within the target heart rate zone, you are in the "aerobic" state (meaning "with oxygen"). During aerobic exercise, like long-distance running, breathing is steady and you can exercise for a long period of time without stopping. When your heart rate is above the zone, like in JONEEBA, you are in an "anaerobic" state (meaning "without oxygen").

JONEEBA!

Steady breathing cannot be maintained for a long period of time without stopping. This is why after a dance routine you will feel winded and need to stop. This type of exercise, such as 100–meter sprints, involves going all out and then resting.

CALORIES

Calories come from food and are used for energy. There are three main sources of calories: fat (such as butter and oil); carbohydrate (such as rice, potatoes and pasta); and protein (such as chicken and red meat). Weight loss occurs when, at the end of the day, the total calories burned off through exercise and daily activity exceed the total calories taken in. If you do the high-intensity exercise involved in JONEEBA for half an hour, you will burn just as many, if not more, calories than if you jog continuously for half an hour. However, in order to reap the optimal fitness benefits from class, including weight loss and maintenance, you need to dance full-out, which means jumping high, lifting your knees all the way up, and swinging your arms out wide.

What is important for staying lean or losing weight through exercise is not that energy burns the fat stored in your body, but how much total energy you use. You will use just as much—if not more—energy in a JONEEBA workout than in a continuous lower-intensity workout, and you will be able to stay lean or lose more weight.

To reap the optimal benefits from class, you need to dance full-out

GETTING THE MOST OUT OF JONEEBA

Carbohydrates are the primary fuel source for energy used in a JONEEBA class. To maintain optimal intensity levels, it is critical to incorporate carbohydrates into your diet through snacks or meals before, during and after dance class.

Approximately 1½ to ½ an hour before class, eat about 50 grams of carbohydrate: the equivalent of half a bagel, a small bowl of pasta or brown rice, a small baked potato, or a Power Bar. Since some people experience side cramps when they eat too soon before exercise, the specific amount of time to leave between eating and class depends on your body. A Snapple or Fresh Samantha are also good sources of both carbohydrate (in the form of fructose) and liquid, which is needed for hydration. Because the sugar in these drinks enters the bloodstream more rapidly, they should be consumed ½ an hour to 5 minutes before class. In a recent study, those who consumed either 50 grams of solid carbohydrate or 50 grams of liquid carbohydrate 5 minutes before exercise were able to sprint 4 minutes longer than those who drank an artificially sweetened solution. Since sprinting uses the same energy system as dance, the consumption of a high-carbohydrate snack before class will prolong dancing ability.

Between consecutive classes, sports drinks such as Gatorade, which contain 4–6 percent carbohydrates (as stated on the label), are recommended. Other quick-energy drinks, such as Snapple, Sprite or orange juice, are also good sources of both carbohydrate and liquid.

After class, the body's carbohydrate stores need to be replenished as quickly as possible. For an optimal rate of refueling, eat a high-carbohydrate snack within two hours. Examples of good refueling snacks or meals are a whole bagel, large bowl of pasta or brown rice, a large baked potato or energy bars such as Cliff, Power, Steel, or MetRx Bars.

PROTEIN AND MUSCLE TONE

The body needs protein not only for muscle tone and strength, but also for other components necessary for athletic performance, such as hemoglobin and myoglobin, which are involved in the flow of oxygen to muscles. Furthermore, as intensity increases in dance class, protein breakdown can increase. Since the body does not store protein in the same way it stores carbohydrates, it is important

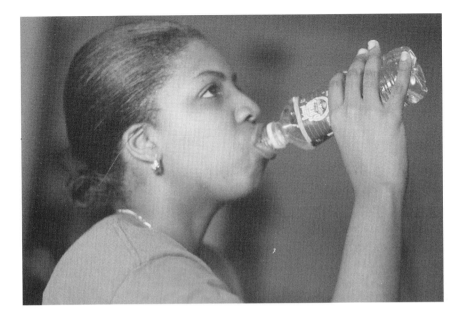

to consume small amounts of high-quality protein throughout the day. Good sources of protein include chicken, turkey, egg whites, fish, non-fat milk and yogurt, soy and whey (commonly found in protein bars).

WATER AND ENERGY

Proper hydration is as important as proper food consumption. During prolonged exercise, including profuse sweating, the body can become dehydrated. Dehydration can impair performance by decreasing endurance, strength and coordination, resulting in feelings of fatigue. When liquid is ingested during exercise, the experience of fatigue is decreased, and exercise can be performed for a longer duration and with more intensity and agility.

To stay hydrated, drink at least eight 8-oz. glasses of water throughout the day. Drink often—not just when you are thirsty. When you feel thirsty, you have already lost important fluids and electrolytes critical not just for dance, but for optimal everyday

Nutrition for Joneeba

functioning. Approximately 2 hours before physical activity, drink at least 2 glasses of water, and during class, drink about 1 glass. (About 2 cups of carbohydrate drink provide the same liquid content as 1 cup of water.) After class, consume 3 glasses of water.

The warning signs of dehydration include dizziness and light-headedness, muscle cramps, nausea and a headache, dark urine, infrequent urination, and a dry mouth and throat. If you notice any of these symptoms during class, take a breather to rehydrate with some cool water.

HUNGER BEFORE CLASS

What should you do when you have barely eaten all day—or at least not as recommended—you are extremely hungry and are about to take a class? It is advisable not to consume a large meal, although that is relative to each individual. Exercise stimulates the sympathetic nervous system, which inhibits parasympathetic processes like digestion. If you exercise on a full stomach, your food will not be completely digested, causing fullness, lethargy, discomfort and stomach cramps. Avoid large meals that are also high in protein and fat. Do not grab a hamburger or slice of pizza, because they take longer to digest and lack the glucose needed for class. Instead, consume a high-carbohydrate meal such as pasta or brown rice, or lower protein energy bars such as a Cliff Bar or Power Bar. Make sure the meal is large enough to satisfy your hunger but not enough to make you totally full. And drink a glass of water, making sure to bring a bottle to class.

OTHER HEALTHY EATING HABITS

The above principles demonstrate how to eat to achieve the maximum fitness benefits from JONEEBA. In addition to pre- and

Table 1

HEALTHY NUTRITION FOR A JONEEBA WORKOUT

Before JONEEBA		During JONEEBA		After JONEEBA
EITHER- 1½ TO ½ HOUR BEFORE	OR ½ HOUR TO 5 MINUTES BEFORE	DURING ONE CLASS	BETWEEN MULTIPLE CLASSES	SOON AFTER
Fluid	**Fluid**	**Fluid**	**Fluid**	**Fluid**
2 cups (16 ounces) of water	*2 cups (16 ounces) of water*	*1 cup (8 ounces) of water*	*At least 1 cup per class with no upper limits*	*3 cups (24 ounces) of water*
Food	**Food**	**Food**	**Food**	**Food**
50 grams of solid carbs Choose one of the following: • Half a bagel • Small bowl of pasta or rice • Small baked potato • Low protein energy bar like a Cliff Bar or Power Bar	*50 grams of liquid carbs* • Snapple If starving: • Choose from examples in first column • Enough to satisfy hunger without becoming too full	*Not advisable*	*45-80 grams of carbs* Choose one of the following: • Gatorade • Snapple • Orange juice • Banana • Low protein energy bar like a Cliff Bar or Power Bar	*80-120 grams of carbs* Choose one of the following: • Whole bagel • Large bowl of pasta or rice • Large baked potato • High protein energy bar like a MetRx or Steel Bar • Low protein energy bar like Cliff Bar or Power Bar

Note: The chart is only a suggestion. You should consult your nutritionist and doctor. People's bodies and metabolism vary greatly. Some people may experience adverse reactions, such as side cramps, when eating close to the exercise session, while others may actually feel better.

Source: Reprinted with permission of the publisher in Robergs, R.A., and Roberts, S.O. (1997). *Exercise Physiology: Exercise, Performance, and Clinical Application.* Boston: Mosby.

post-dance eating habits, other nutrition pointers are equally important for weight loss, weight maintenance, and energy enhancement. Although a complete nutrition prescription is beyond the scope of this book, here are some suggestions:

- ꙮ Rather than three large meals, eat five or six small meals throughout the day. A certain amount of energy is used to metabolize food, so spreading out your meals this way can actually speed up your metabolism.

- ꙮ Complement your diet with vitamin and mineral supplements, but do not use them in place of food.

- ꙮ Choose whole grains, such as brown rice and whole-wheat bread because they contain more nutrients and less sugar than refined grains. Consumption of high-sugar foods causes an immediate burst of energy followed by fatigue, unless you exercise soon after eating the high-sugar food.

- ꙮ Decrease your intake of saturated fat, such as butter and red meat. Also decrease your intake of hydrogenated oil, an ingredient in margarine and products like potato chips. These fats lead not just to weight gain, but more importantly, to heart disease. Replace saturated and hydrogenated fats with the ones found in fish such as tuna and salmon; nuts such as flaxseed; and vegetable oils. However, make sure to refrigerate vegetable oils so they do not become rancid, or hydrogenated, from exposure to oxygen and heat.

- ꙮ Drink alcohol moderately or not at all. Drinking will sabotage your exercise and healthy eating habits, diminishing energy and preventing the body from burning off fat.

Use these nutrition suggestions in accordance with your nutritionist and physician not only to optimize your JONEEBA class, but also to build and maintain a healthy, strong and beautiful body!

CHAPTER 10

INJURY PREVENTION

The human body is more complex than the most advanced technologies. Therefore, your body must be treated like the valuable machine it is. You have approximately 635 muscles and 206 bones, which make up about 15% of your body weight. To gain all of the benefits that a JONEEBA class provides, proper basic nutrition is necessary. Equally important is proper maintenance of the muscular and skeletal systems. The basic things that can be done to provide appropriate care for the muscular and skeletal systems will be considered in this chapter.

MAINTENANCE AND PREVENTION

If you are starting an exercise program, begin slowly and gradually increase the intensity in order to allow your muscular and skeletal systems to grow based on the demands of the exercise and to decrease your risk of injury. It is normal to have a slight amount of soreness when beginning a new program.

Because the muscular and skeletal systems are used on an average of 10–12 hours per day for many different types of activities, they need to be well maintained to prevent breakdown. Here are the best ways to do so.

WARM UP AND COOL DOWN

It is important to do the exercises and stretches of the warm-up in the order provided to thoroughly prepare the body for the high-intensity workout. After a JONEEBA class, it is recommended to perform further stretching to help increase the length of muscles, decrease any soreness and maintain healthy muscles.

AVOIDING INJURIES

The most common muscle and skeletal injuries are sprains, bruises and strains. If you suffer an injury, stop exercising immediately. Do not try to work through the pain or ignore it. Pain is your body's way

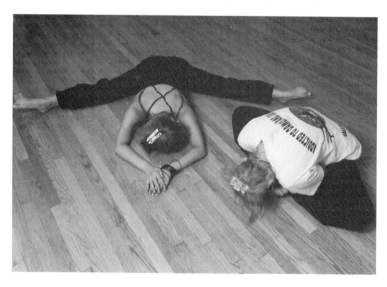

of telling you that something is wrong. Ignoring and working through pain is similar to turning off a smoke alarm that has gone off in your house in the middle of the night and then going back to sleep without further investigation.

The injured person should find

a position of comfort. Apply ice to the area for no longer than fifteen minutes. Do not apply heat under any circumstances! Why? Because the body has a natural healing process called tissue repair that occurs in response to injury. During the course of tissue repair, the body makes chemicals that cause pain and attract cells that destroy tissue in the area of the injury. This process is called inflammation. The tissue repair and inflammatory process is the exact and precise amount needed to heal naturally, not more. Applying heat will over-increase the repair and inflammatory process, causing greater pain, discomfort, tissue damage and prolonged healing time. After an injury, it is wise to seek the care of a doctor skilled in the treatment of athletic injuries immediately.

*Pain is your body's way of
telling you that something
is wrong*

PART IV
IT'S JONEEBA! TIME

HEAR THE RHYTHM...

NOW LET THE DRUMS

FREE YOUR MIND

FOLLOW THE SPIRIT

IT'S JONEEBA! TIME.

CHAPTER 11

THE WARM-UP

Since 1984, I have used a warm-up routine that I developed to prepare you for any ethnic dance class. It has received a lot of praise for its fast, effective results. It also has served as a model for many teachers who use either a portion of or the entire routine in their classes.

The warm-up is designed for optimal fitness benefits: strength, flexibility and injury prevention for high-intensity dancing. It begins with some simple exercises that initiate blood flow to the muscles so they receive oxygen and other vital nutrients to perform optimally. It continues with stretching and more calisthenics that stretch and strengthen all the muscle groups. The stretching exercises come second, because studies show that gains in flexibility are achieved only after muscles are already warm. Then, during the high-intensity part, not only do your muscles become stronger, but so does your heart, improving its use of energy.

The exercises loosen up the entire body, from the head, neck and shoulders down to the toes. Isolations are important here because they will be sped up into full movements once the dancing begins. It is important to get in touch with each part of the body before dancing because JONEEBA movements are fluid and comprehensive—every part of the body moves to create the whole movement. The JONEEBA warm-up is always used in every class. It is uninterrupted and designed to allow anyone from beginners to advanced dancers to follow easily.

STRETCHING

JONEEBA is a rigorous class, and the body needs to prepare itself for the movement. The best way to do this is through a good warm-up, which means breathing deeply and stretching so that the muscles are limber and ready to move and dance when the time comes. In Africa, I've witnessed many an impromptu circle gather quickly around drummers and watched as pedestrians and people who were just hanging around suddenly answered the drums with explosive dancing. Arms swinging, hips shaking, legs whirling, feet jumping. The drums just lit them up.

Did they do a quick set of knee raises, some lunges and head isolations before coming over to the crowd? Did they do 50 jumping jacks to warm up their bodies? Or maybe a few shoulder rolls and a couple of knee bends? No. The warm climate and the sun keep the muscles limber. Also, most people would jump into the circle for a signature moment to execute one or two steps at a time without straining themselves—not for a 1½-hour-long dance workout.

Western culture, on the other hand, is very sedentary. People drive a lot and they sit for long periods of time. Many don't work out at all. In Africa, people still get much of their exercise by walking long distances. In most of the United States, the weather is much colder than in West Africa. Colder weather and sedentary lifestyles are good reasons to really give our bodies a chance to warm up.

Stretching before an intense workout helps warm the muscles, which makes them more flexible and decreases the chances of injury.

When you stretch or dance, you should not disregard any sign of pain or discomfort. Pain is the body's way of telling you to be on the alert and slow down.

BREATHING

Breathing is an integral part of life and especially important when you work out. Deep breathing helps push oxygen from the lungs to the blood. By supplying more oxygen, the body feels better and more alive.

Studying Hatha yoga, a system of exercises that combines various postures and stretches with deep breathing, helped me appreciate the important combination of breathing and stretching. Proper breathing when you stretch or exercise can be done in different combinations.

If you really want to focus on deep-breathing techniques, then you should try to fill up your belly first and then your chest with air, and then exhale until your body is empty. You can inhale on the stretching and exhale on the release. In my experience, I have realized that people either focus too much on breathing or forget to breathe at all. So I suggest the middle ground. That means remembering to breathe all the time by taking in as much air as you can and pushing out as much as you can. Of course, the faster you do a movement, the less air you can take in and out. The important thing is just to remember to breathe!

And here's a tip I learned in Africa from the national ballet. When you actually start dancing, keep your mouth open and wear a big smile. There is a two-fold reason for this. First, keeping your mouth open forces you to remember to breathe through your nose and your mouth. And showing those pearly whites puts a positive energy on your face that filters throughout your body.

FINDING YOUR CENTER

The abdomen is one the most difficult areas of the body to keep fit and strengthen. It is from this area that everything emanates. It is also where you find your balance. A large portion of the JONEEBA warm-up is designed to work on the abdominal area. If this area is weak, then your dancing will also be weak. You won't be able to lift your legs high, jump, or bend your body in certain ways.

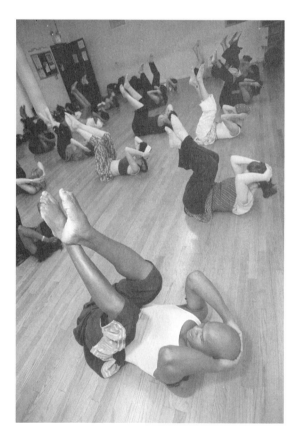

CHAPTER 12

THE EXERCISES

START-UP

12.1—SPINE ROLLS

Place your feet together in parallel hip width apart (1). Start rolling your body down, head first (2). Go down as far as you can, keeping your legs straight (3–4). Then roll back up, with the head coming up last. Use each vertebra in the spine as you roll down and up. Count of 8 down, count of 8 up. (4x)

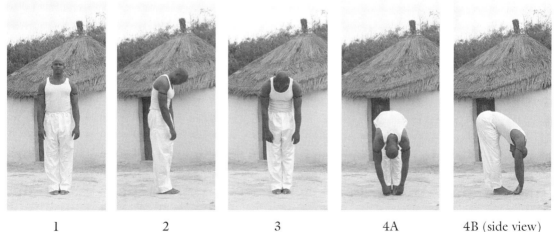

| 1 | 2 | 3 | 4A | 4B (side view) |

12.2—PLIES (KNEE BENDS)

Place your feet together parallel (1). With your spine straight and stomach pulled in, bend the knees, arms to side (2), then stand, arms down (3). With arms swinging overhead, lift the heels while standing on the balls of your feet, being sure to keep the knees straight (4), then lower the heels flat back to parallel position with arms open (5). Keeping your arms open and spine straight, go into a deep bend of the knees all the way down, allowing the heels to lift off the floor (6), then slowly return to standing position (7). Do this for 8 counts. (4x)

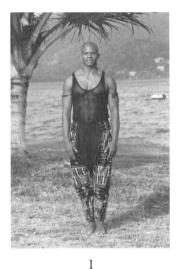

1

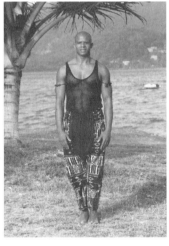

2

3

JONEEBA!

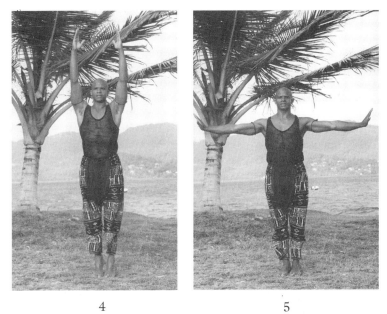

4   5

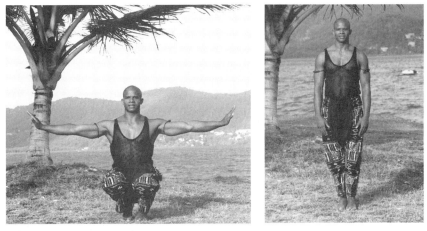

6   7

The Exercises

12.3—CALVES / FEET STRETCH

Place your feet together parallel. With your spine straight, lift both heels (1), then lower left heel and bend right knee (2). Lift up both heels (3), then lower right heel while bending left knee (4). Lift one heel, then lower while alternating sides. This will give you a good calf stretch and warm up the feet. Do this exercise gently. (16x)

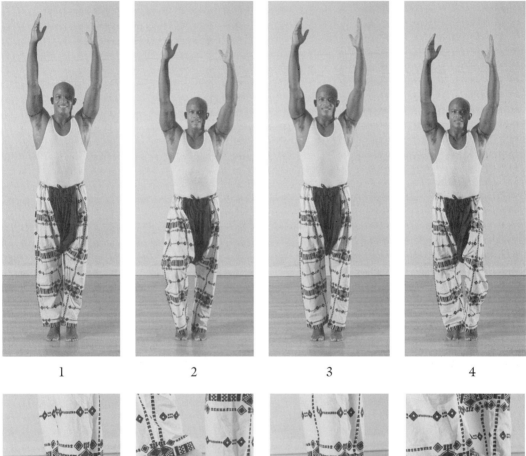

| 1 | 2 | 3 | 4 |

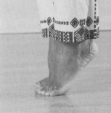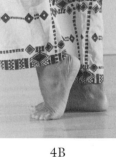

| 1B | 2B | 3B | 4B |

JONEEBA!

12.4—SPINE ROTATION

Place your feet in a wide second position. With your spine straight, place hands behind your head (1). Rotate to the right (2), then left (3) at the hip. Be sure to keep your knees straight and your pelvis fixed. (8x)

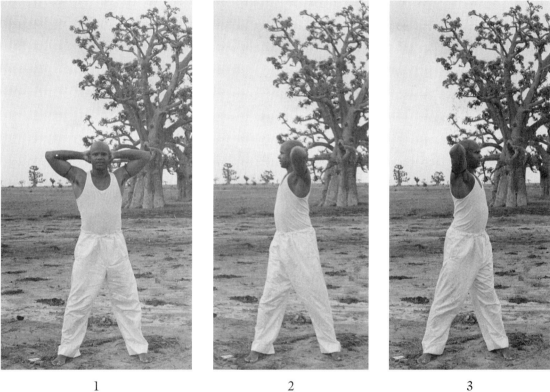

1   2   3

12.5A—SIDE LUNGES

Step right foot to the side, lifting right knee directly into lunge. Your arms should be stretched to the sides with your torso facing front (1). Then lift left knee high to lunge to the left, with arms coming in to the chest, clapping hands together (2). (8x)

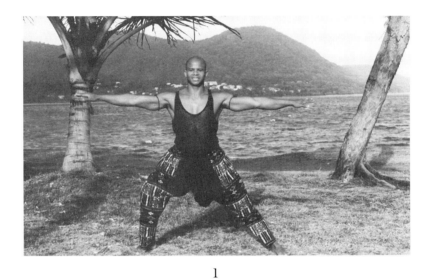

1

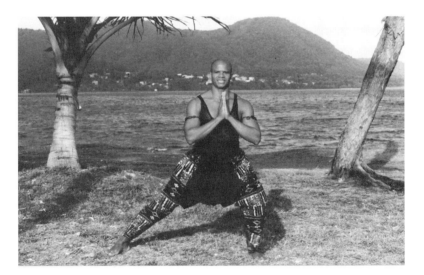

2

12.5B—DEEP LUNGES

Open your feet in wide second position (1). Lunge to the right, placing your hands on the floor (2–3). Begin to stand, bringing arms up in a circle (4). Come to a standing position, lifting arms in a circle (5–6). Lunge to the left, placing your hands on the floor again (7), then stand, bringing arms overhead in a circle (8–9).

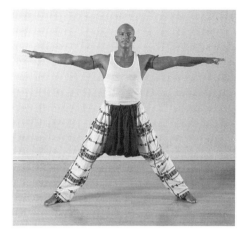

1

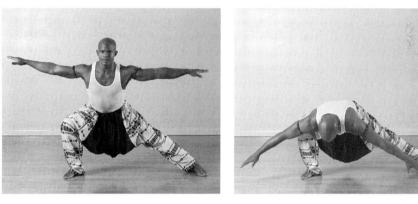

2   3

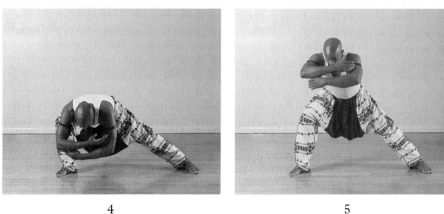

4   5

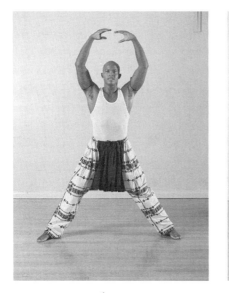

6

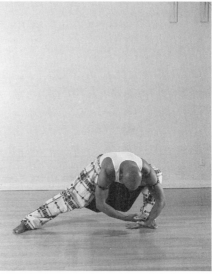

7

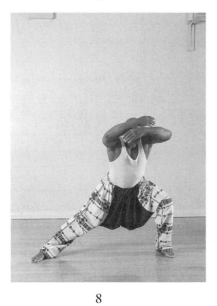

8

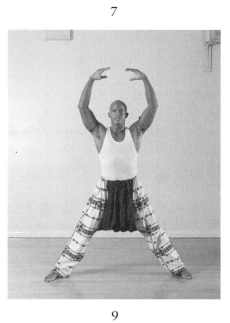

9

JONEEBA!

12.6—LATERAL SERIES

Open feet in second position, with arms out to the sides (1). Reach body and right arm to the right (2). Reach left arm to the right, keeping your torso open and flat to the front. Legs are straight (3). Turn torso to the side, facing the floor with a flat back and reaching both arms out (4). Pull torso down toward the right leg and hold the position (5). Then move torso to the center of the body, facing the floor. Grab both ankles if you can (6). Roll up, with head coming up last (7–8). Repeat to left side (9–10–11–12–13–14–15). (4x)

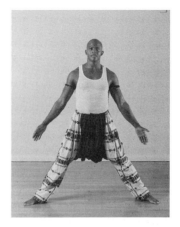

1

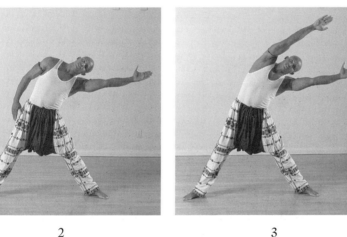

2   3

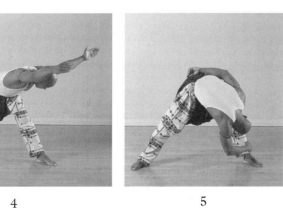

4   5   6

The Exercises

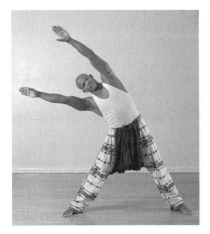

7

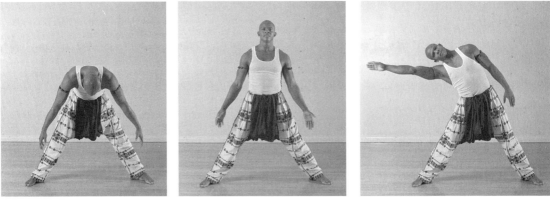

8

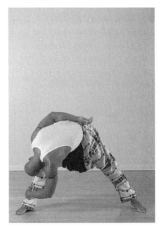

9

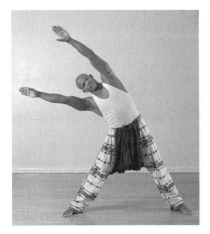

10

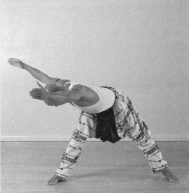

11

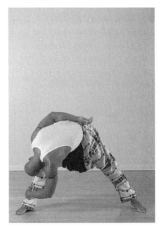

12

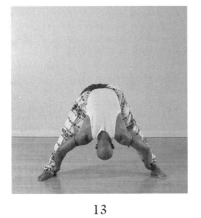

13

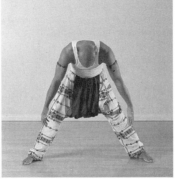

14

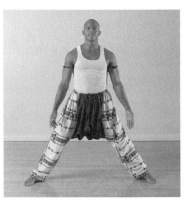

15

JONEEBA!

12.7—BACK STRETCH

Keep feet open in parallel second position with arms at sides (1). Slowly lift arms in front of the body and overhead, stretching the torso up and arching your back (2–3). Then return body to upright position (4) and slowly lower the arms down in front of body (5) and back to sides (6). (4x)

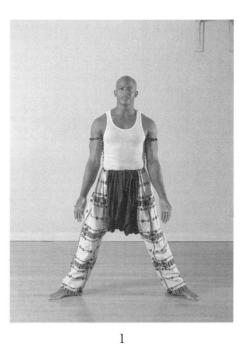

1

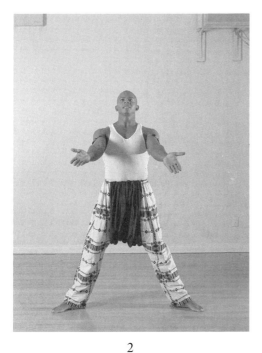

2

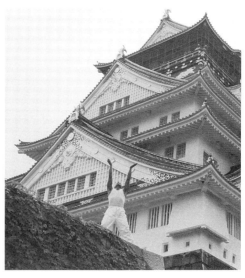

3

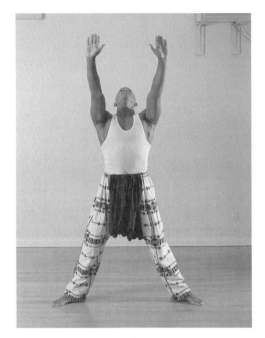

4

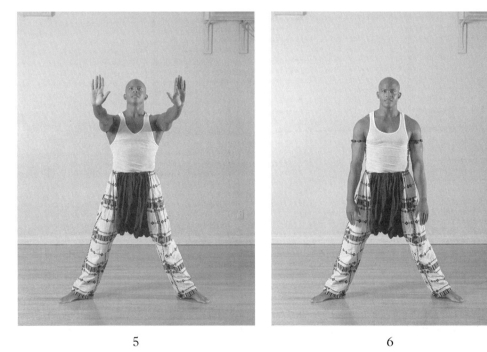

5

6

JONEEBA!

12.8—PLIE & LUNGE

Start with your feet together in a full squat with your heels off the floor. With your spine straight, stomach in, and arms front (1), place your right leg behind in a lunge position, with your chest leaning forward. Hands are on the floor on either side of the front foot (2). With your hands still on the floor, bring back your right leg into a squatting position with feet together and heels off the floor (3). Then place your right leg back a second time in a lunge position for a full stretch (4). Bring your right leg in a second time into a squatting position (5). Repeat the exercise with your left leg (2–3–4). Then go back into a full squat position (5). Grab your ankles or toes and straighten your knees, touching your knees with your head if you're able (6). Repeat exercise from (1). (2x)

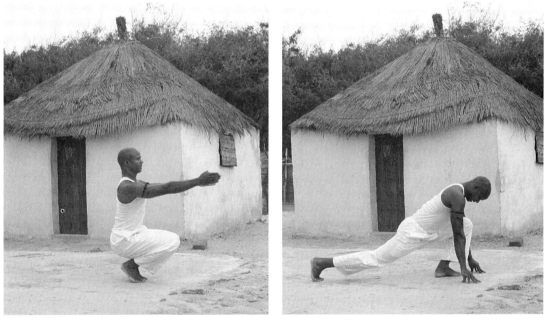

1   2

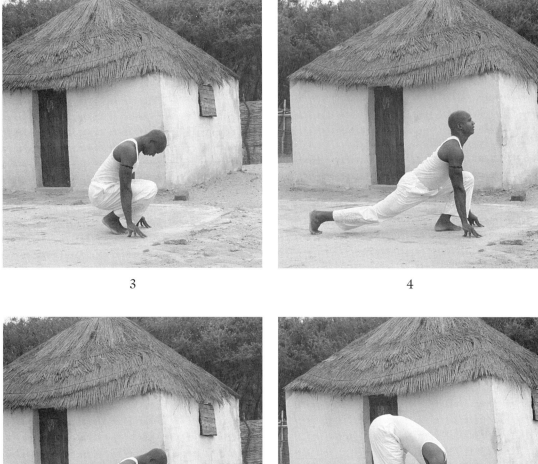

3

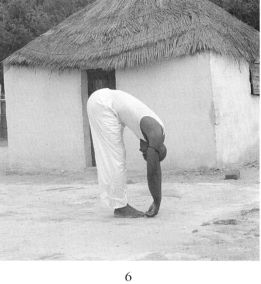

4

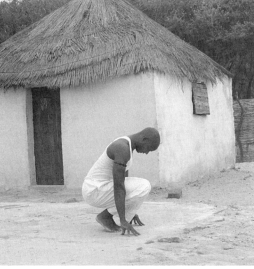

5

6

12.9—PARALLEL WALK

Start with your feet together parallel bending your torso over (1). Step forward with your right foot. Gently bounce your torso up and down, touching the floor with your hands while keeping your knees straight to stretch the back of your legs (2). Step forward with your left foot, gently bouncing up (3) and down (4), putting hands on the floor to stretch the legs. Walk forward 8 steps and backward 8 steps. (2x)

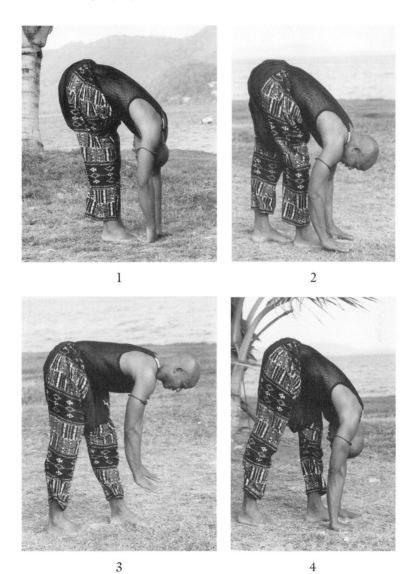

1   2

3   4

FLOOR SEQUENCE

12.10—BACK ARCH

Kneel in upright position, keeping your pelvis straight (1). Open your arms to the side (2). Arch your back, lifting your chest, and tilt your head back while closing your arms in front of your torso. Be sure to keep your pelvis up and facing forward (3–4–5). Slowly return to original position (6–7). (4x)

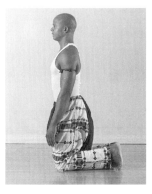

1

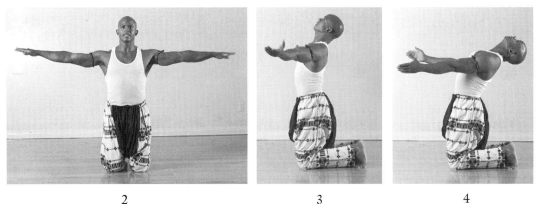

2   3   4

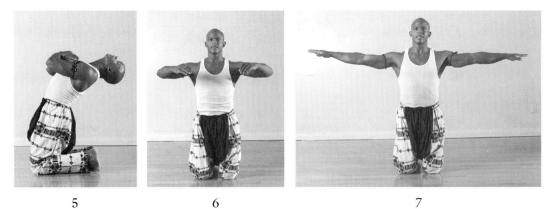

5   6   7

12.11—SEMI-BRIDGE

Start with your arms up, kneeling down with your torso and chest up (1) while moving to the right into a sitting position (2). With feet at least hip width apart, place right hand behind back on the floor and left arm in front of the body (3). Push pelvis straight up and straighten left arm to the ceiling (4). Return to seated position, switching arms behind back (5). Repeat on other side with left hand behind you. (3–4–5)

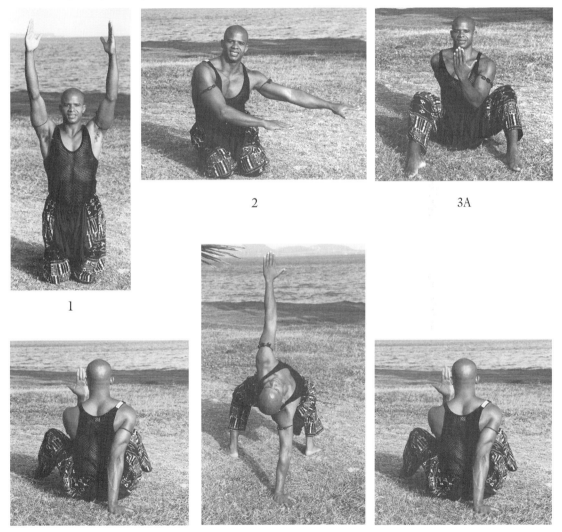

1

2

3A

3B (Back view)

4

5

12.12—BRIDGE

Start with your hands up while sitting upright with knees bent, feet on the floor at least hip width apart (1). Lie on your back with arms just over shoulders near the ears. Place hands flat on the floor (2–3). Push up pelvis (4) and back as high as possible with head arched fully backward (5). Stay in that position for 16 counts while breathing deeply with long inhalations and exhalations. Lower back and pelvis and lie on the floor (6–7).

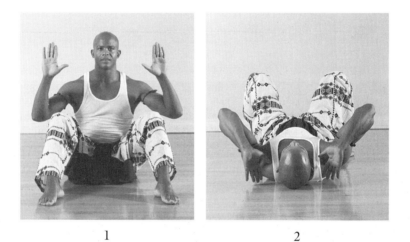

| 1 | 2 |

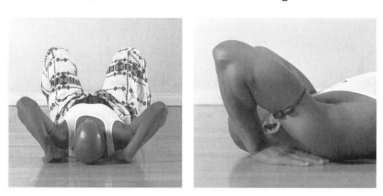

| 3A | 3B (Close-up) |

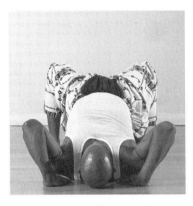

4B

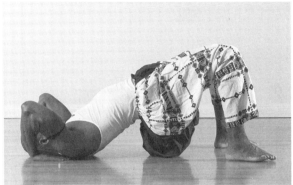

4B (Side view)

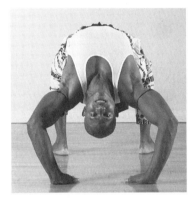

5A

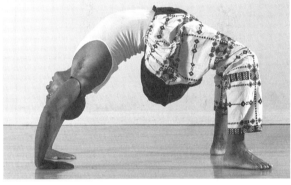

5B (Side view)

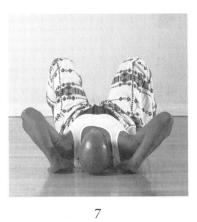

6

7

The Exercises

12.13—WAIST & ANKLE STRETCH

Lie on back with legs straight in air above the hips, and stretch arms out in front of the torso (1). Roll hands and feet in circles (2–3). (8x)

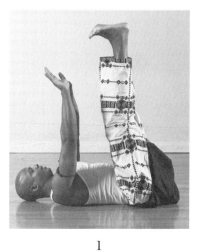

1

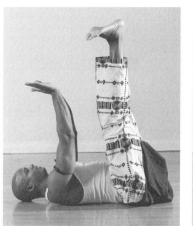

2

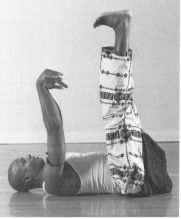

3

12.14—THIGH & FEET STRETCH

Stretch your legs out to the side, holding and pressing down on your straight knees. Then point the feet (1), and flex them (2). (8x)

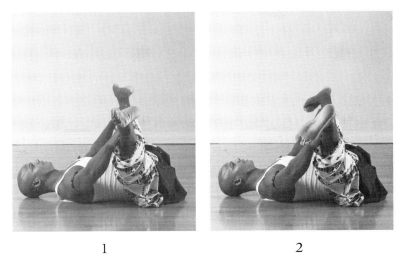

1   2

12.15—ABDOMEN CRUNCHES

Lie on your back with your legs stretched up in the air. Your hands should be down by your hips (1). Bend your knees in toward your chest while lifting your head off the floor and looking front (2). Then straighten your knees and legs to the front in a 45° angle, keeping your lower back on the floor (3). Bend your knees back toward your chest while keeping your head off the floor (4). Then repeat. (16x)

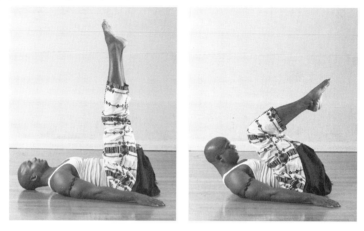

1   2

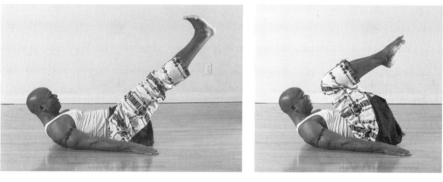

3   4

12.16—THIGH & FEET STRETCH
Repeat exercise 12.14 to prepare for abdomen crunches.

12.17— ABDOMEN CRUNCHES
Repeat exercise 12.15 to complete abdomen crunch sequence.

JONEEBA!

12.18—CANOE SIT-UPS

Lie on your back with knees bent, feet flat on the floor and arms at your sides (1). Raise your head off the ground and look forward. Roll up from your head and bring your torso into an upright position (2), bringing your hands in toward your chest (3). Lean forward and push your arms out (4). Then recline, circling your arms inward as though you were rowing back into the starting position (5–6–7–8) with your head slightly off the ground looking forward (9). Repeat. (8x–16x)

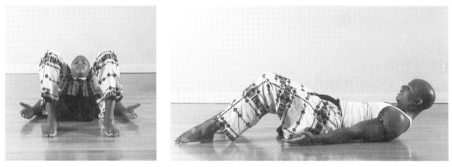

1A   1B (Side view)

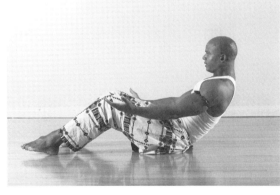 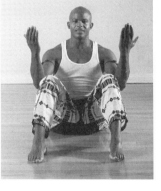

2   3

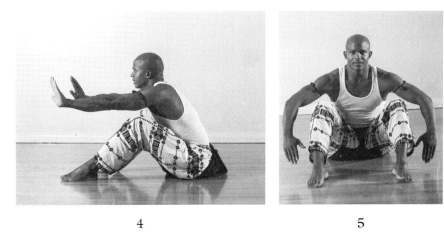

4   5

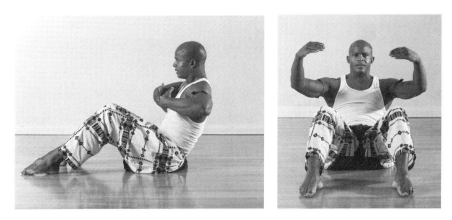

6   7

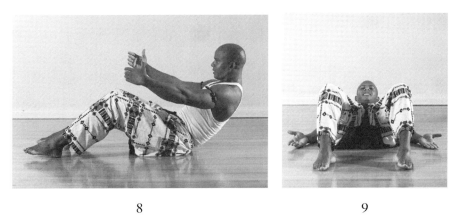

8   9

JONEEBA!

12.19—LEG LIFTS

Keeping your feet on the floor and arms straight up overhead, bend your knees (1). Keeping your spine straight, straighten and raise your right leg (2) then lower leg slightly without allowing it to touch the floor (3). Repeat 2 & 3. (16x) Next, bend both legs with your feet on the floor to rest. Grab the knees with your hands and pull your chest forward while breathing slow and deep (4–5). Then repeat with the left leg (6). (16x)

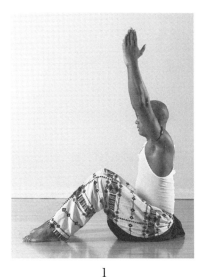

1

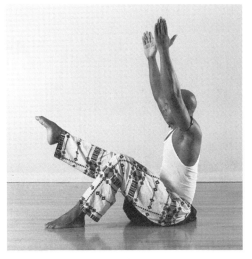

2A

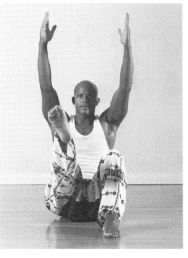

2B (Front view)

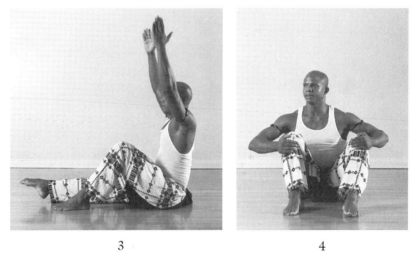

3

4

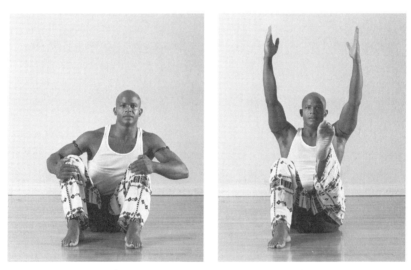

5

6

JONEEBA!

12.20—ARM STAND

While lying on your back, bring your knees toward your chest and rock backwards wrapping your arms around your thighs for support (1–2). Place elbows on the floor and put your hands on either side of your waist. Lift your legs in a vertical position, with weight resting on the shoulders (3–4–5). Stay in that position for 16 counts while inhaling and exhaling deeply. Lower your legs back toward your head (6) and let your toes touch the floor outstretched over the head (7). Place your arms on the floor for support (8). Stay in that position for 16 counts while inhaling and exhaling deeply. Roll forward into a sitting second position (9–10–11).

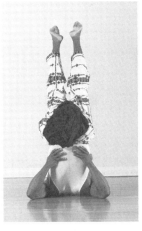

1

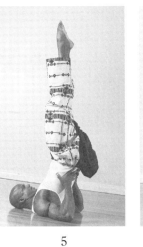

2

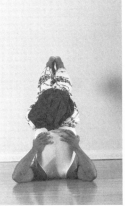

3

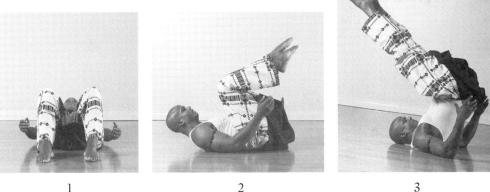

4

5

6

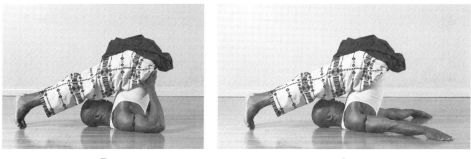

7

8

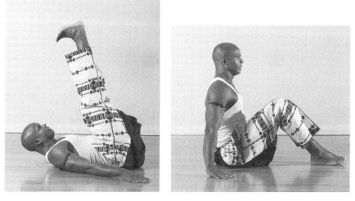

9

10

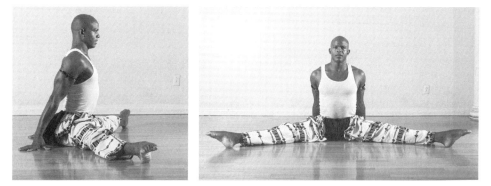

11A

11B (Front view)

JONEEBA!

12.21—DEEP-SECOND STRETCH

Sitting with your legs open in a wide second position, bend your torso forward and rest head and arms in front of you. Relax the hip joints and thigh muscles. Don't forget to take deep breaths. (8 counts)

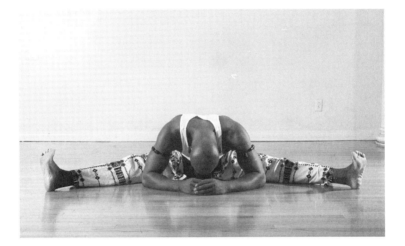

 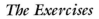

12.22—SECOND POSITION STRETCH

Start in a wide second position with your back straight (1). Reach to the left side with your right arm overhead, keeping your shoulders open and chest lifted up to the ceiling (2). (8x) Repeat on the other side, reaching left arm overhead to the right (3). (8x) Return to center (4–5) and gently stretch forward with both arms outstretched in second (6). (8x) Repeat (2–3–4–5–6) in decreasing counts. (4x, 2x, then 1x)

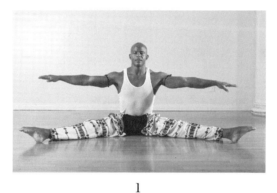

1

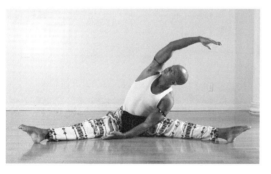

2

3

JONEEBA!

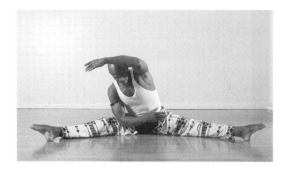

4

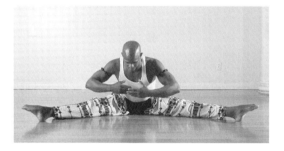

5

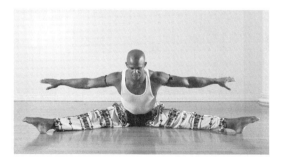

6

12.23—STRAIGHT LEG BACK STRETCH

Bring legs together in front of you, keeping the knees straight. If flexibility allows, hold your feet and stretch forward with your head down toward your knees while taking deep breaths. (8 counts) If you cannot reach your feet, hold onto your ankles or shins.

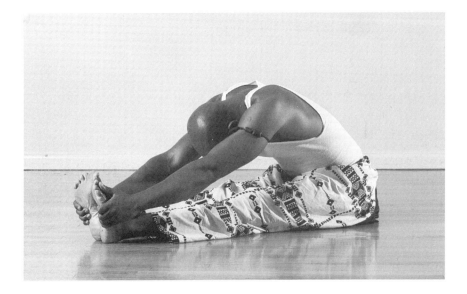

12.24—CROSSED LEG CRUNCHES

Face the back of the room. Lie on your back with your legs bent and feet on floor. Bring knees toward the chest and put hands behind head. Contract abdomen, bringing your elbows to your knees. Your head should not touch the floor. Do not lift your head with your hands; use them only for support. The contraction should be short and fast (1–2). Repeat twice. (16x each)

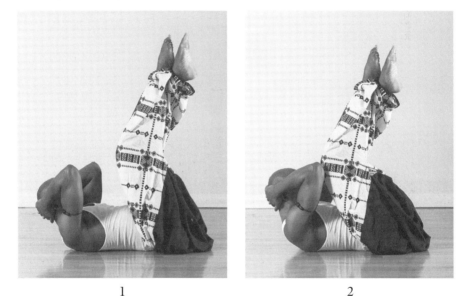

1   2

12.25—TRANSITION
(from Crunches to Cobra)

Lie on your back with your arms at your sides. Raise your head off the floor (1). Turn to your right onto your chest (2–3).

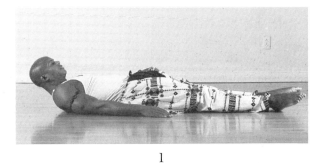

1

2

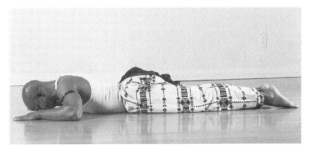

3

12.26—COBRA

Lie on floor face down. With arms beside shoulders (1), push upper body up until arms and elbows are straight, leaving hips on the floor. Keep shoulders down (2–3). Bend arms and lower torso to floor (4).

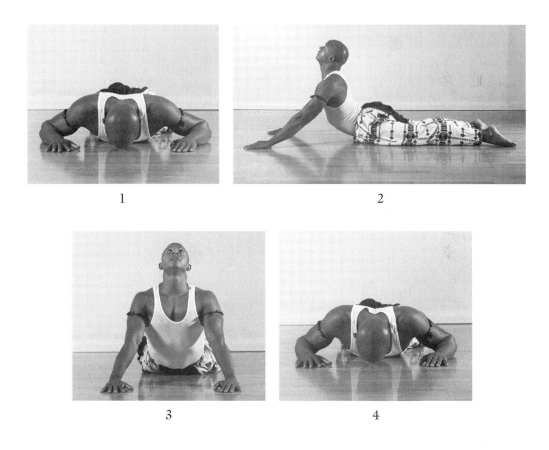

1

2

3

4

12.27—PLANE

Lie on the floor face down with your hands next to your head. Slowly raise your legs, contracting your buttock muscles (1). Slowly raise straight arms and chest, contracting your back muscles while keeping your legs raised (2). Open arms to the back beside your body, slowly raising the torso with arms extended back (3). Release and return to resting position (4–6).

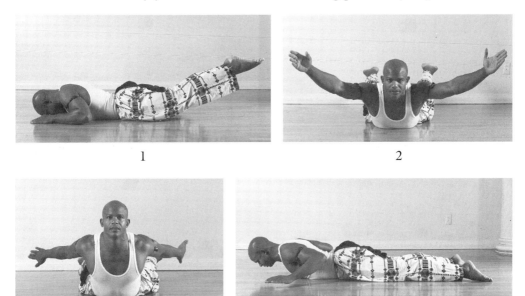

1

2

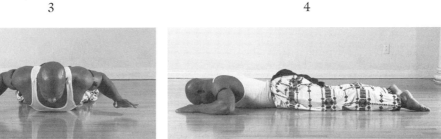

3

4

5

6

12.28—COBRA
Repeat exercise 12.26.
12.29—PLANE
Repeat exercise 12.27.

12.30—BACK STRETCH

Lie face down on the floor, hands on the floor at chest level. (1) Come up to your knees, keeping hands on the floor and back straight. (2) Sit back on the calves, stretching out the arms and back with your head resting on floor (3).

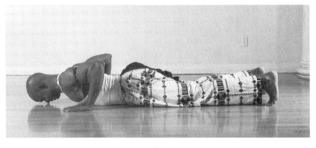

1

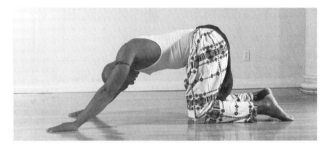

2

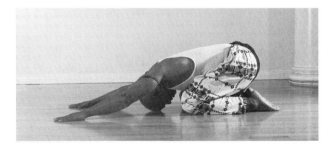

3

 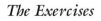

12.31—BACK CONTRACTIONS

On hands and knees, keep elbows straight and curl toes down against the floor. (1) Contract torso, tuck head and look down (2). Release, curve torso and head and look up (3). Repeat. (8x)

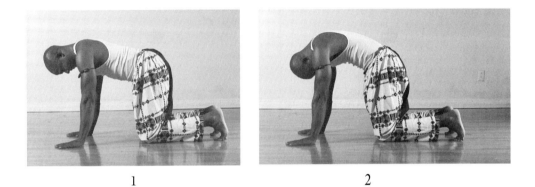

1   2

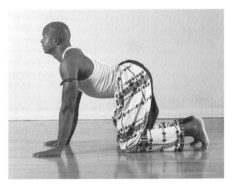

3

12.32— LEG KICK (BACK)

On hands and knees, extend right leg back as far as you can (1). Raise your right leg higher, keeping arms and right knee straight (2). Do not lower your leg past the starting position (3). Repeat (1–2–3). (16x) Then bring right leg into floor, moving into a back stretch position (4). Return to hands and knees and repeat (1–2–3) with left leg back. (16x)

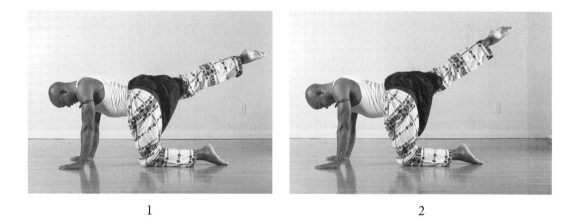

1

2

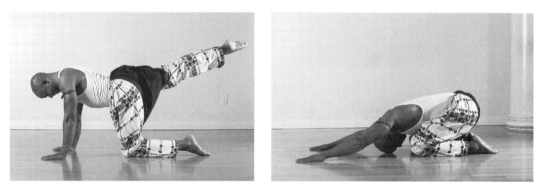

3

4

12.33— LEG KICK (Side)

Raise bent right leg to side and raise your leg and knee up (1) and down (2). (16x) Be sure not to kick front and back. The movement should be up and down (3). Then, move into back stretch position to rest (4). Switch to the left leg and repeat exercise. (16x)

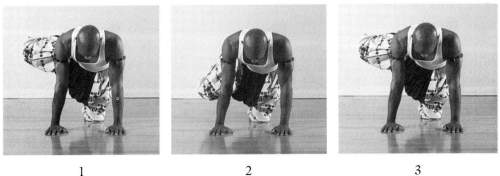

1   2   3

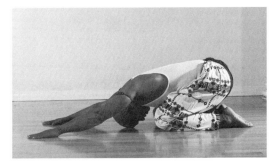

4

JONEEBA!

12.34—CALF STRETCH

Place hands and feet on the floor a couple of feet apart until heels feel like they want to come off the floor. Legs and arms are straight and hips should be the highest point. Keep shoulders and head down (1). Press left heel into the floor, stretching the left calf (2). Then come back up, both heels off floor (3) and lower right heel, stretching right calf (4). (8x)

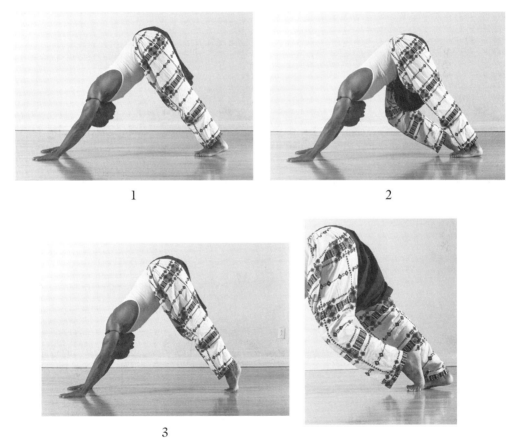

1

2

3

4

12.35—MEN'S PUSH-UP

Lie on the floor face down. Place your hands flat on the floor parallel to your shoulders (1). Use your arms to lift entire body off the floor (2). (16x)

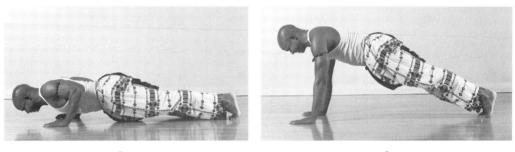

1   2

12.36—WOMEN'S PUSH-UP

Lie on the floor face down. Place your hands flat on floor parallel to your shoulders (1). Place your knees on the floor, keeping your hips straight. Use your arms to gradually lift upper half of your body off floor (2). (16x)

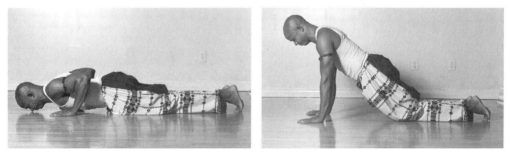

1   2

ISOLATIONS

12.37—HEAD ISOLATION

Start standing with feet parallel and open shoulder width apart. Place your hands on your hips and look right (1), then left (2). Repeat (8x). Look down (3), then up (4). Repeat (8x). Tilt head right (5), then left (6). Repeat (8x). Move head (2x around) to the right, rolling head down (7–8), right (9–10), back (11), and left. Reverse head roll (2x) to the left, rolling down, left, back, and right.

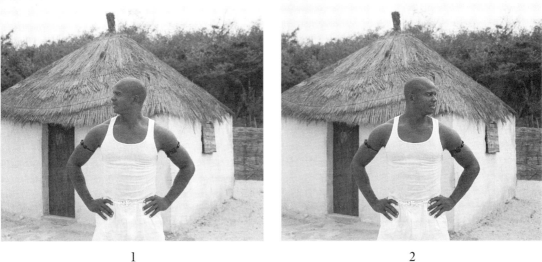

1   2

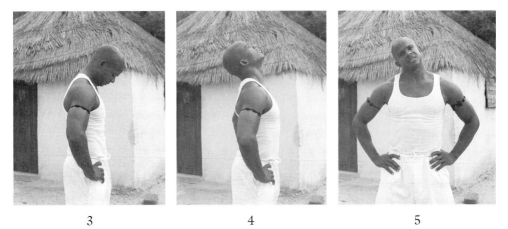

3　　　　　　　4　　　　　　　5

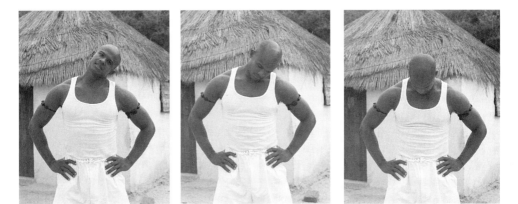

6　　　　　　　7　　　　　　　8

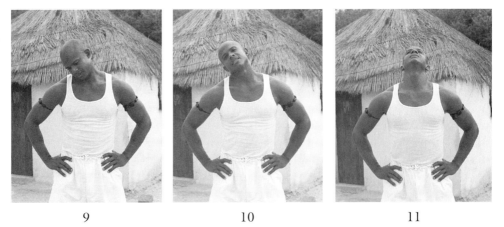

9　　　　　　　10　　　　　　11

JONEEBA!

12.38—CHEST ISOLATION

Place hands on hips and stretch shoulder to the right (1), then left (2). Do (8x) slowly. Then push chest forward (3), and contract it back (4). Do (8x). Then repeat right and left faster (8x). Then, repeat front and back faster (8x).

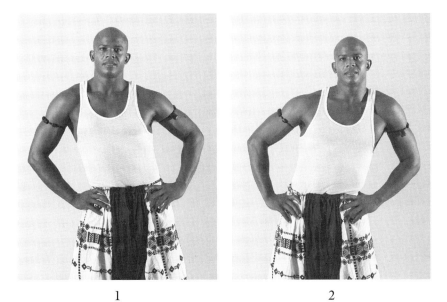

1   2

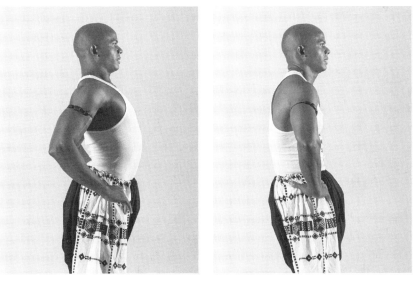

3   4

12.39—DEEP CONTRACTION

Place hands on shoulders, pushing out and releasing chest forward and inhaling (1). Bend the knees, extend the arms forward while contracting the chest back (2). While keeping your knees bent, bring arms down to the hips and release the chest forward (3). Repeat #2, (4) then repeat #1. (5) (4x) Keep the same breathing pattern throughout the exercise: exhale with the contraction and inhale with release.

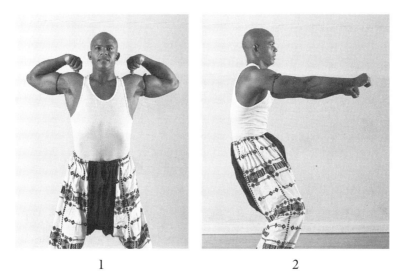

1   2

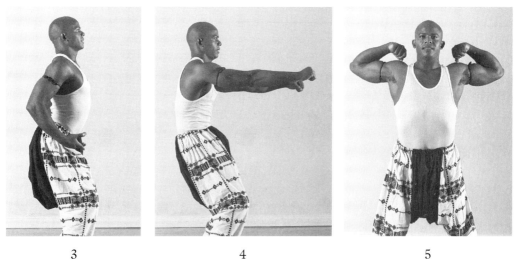

3   4   5

JONEEBA!

12.40—FAST CONTRACTION

Bend the knees and extend the arms forward while contracting the chest back (1).
While keeping your knees bent, bend arms back and release the chest forward (2).
Repeat (3–4). (16x) Be sure to keep your knees bent throughout the exercise. Also,
keep the same breathing pattern throughout the exercise: exhale with the contraction and inhale with the release.

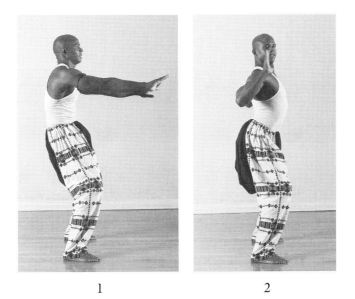

1 2

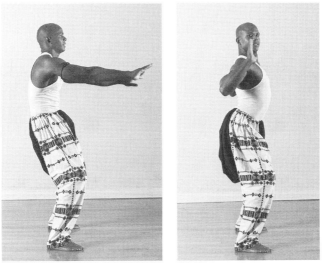

3 4

12.41—HIP ISOLATION
(SIDE, FRONT, BACK)

Side: Bend knees, move hips from center to the right (1), (8x) then from center to the left (2). (8x) **Front:** Move hips from center (3) to front switching right arm (4), and left arm (5) every 2 counts (8x). **Back:** With both arms front and hands dropped, move hips from center (6) to back while flexing hands (7). (8x)

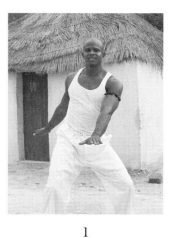

1

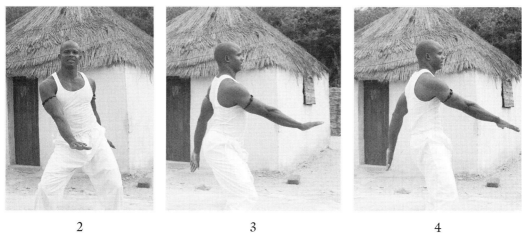

2   3   4

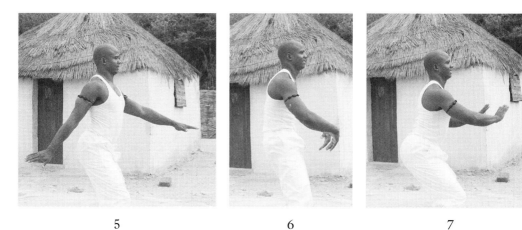

5   6   7

12.42—HIP ROLL (UP / DOWN, AROUND)

With your knees bent, roll your hips around in a circular motion to the right (1), front (2), left (3), and back (4), clapping your hands every two rolls. (8 rolls)

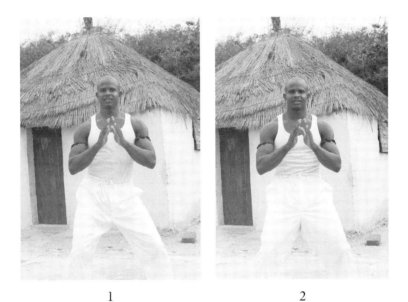

1   2

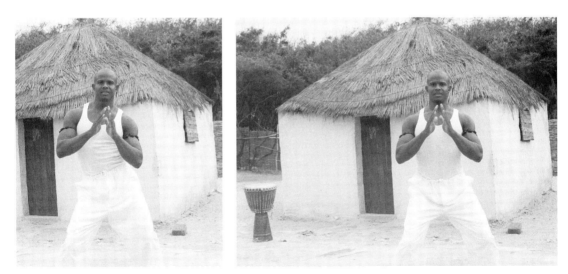

3   4

12.43—SHOULDER ISOLATION (UP / DOWN, AROUND)

Up / Down: Lift shoulders up toward ears (1), release them down (2). (8x)
Around: Circle shoulder from front (3) to upward position (4) to back (5) to
down position (6). (8x) Reverse the circle with shoulders from back, to upward
position, front, and down (5–4–3–2) (8x).

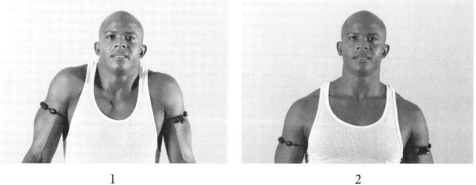

1	2

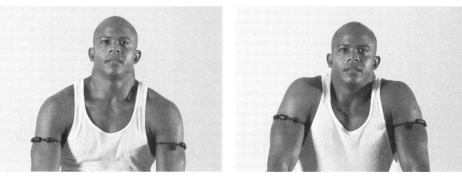

3	4

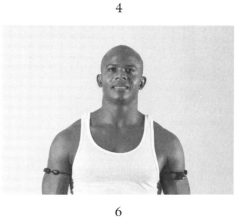

5	6

JONEEBA!

JUMPS

12.44—STRAIGHT JUMP

This jump will prepare you and warm you up for the more difficult jumps in exercises 12.45 and 12.46. Start in standing position with feet slightly open and parallel while bending your knees (1) and push off floor keeping your body and knees straight (2). Land like a cat, bending into the floor and using your knees and feet like a spring and cushion (3). Bending your knees is important when landing to ease the shock. (4x)

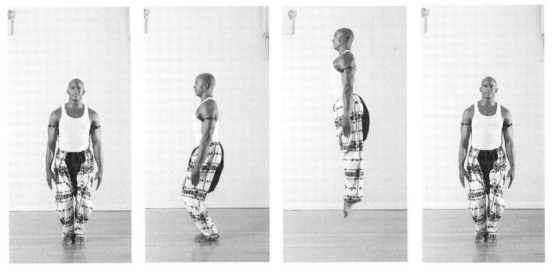

| 1A | 1B (Side view) | 2 | 3 |

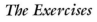

12.45—KNEES TO CHEST (WITHOUT ARMS)

Bend your knees with hands down at your side (1). Push off floor with legs, bringing your knees to your chest with arms remaining down (2). Land like a cat, bending and using your knees and feet like a spring (3). (4x)

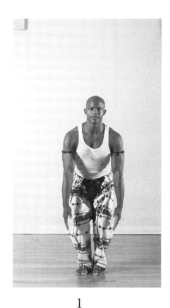

1

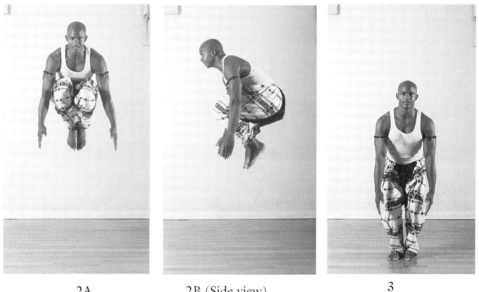

2A   2B (Side view)   3

12.46—KNEES TO CHEST (WITH ARMS)

Bend your knees with hands to your chest (1). Push off floor with legs, bringing your knees to your chest while opening and swinging your arms to the side to give you more momentum to jump high (2). Land like a cat, bending and using your knees and feet like a spring and cushion (3). (4x)

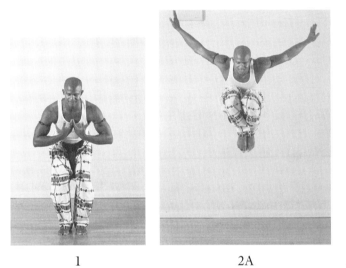

1   2A

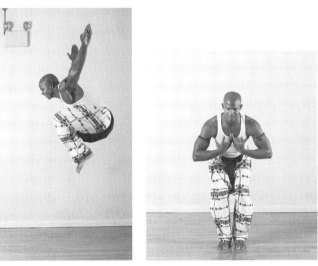

2B (Side view)   3

12.47—ADVANCED STRADDLE JUMP

Start in standing position with feet slightly open and parallel while bending your knees (1). Push off floor, opening and kicking both legs to the side. Slightly lean torso forward. Swing your arms to the side to help you pull your body into the air (2). Land like a cat, bending and using your knees and feet like a springboard or cushion (3). (4x)

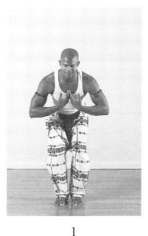

1

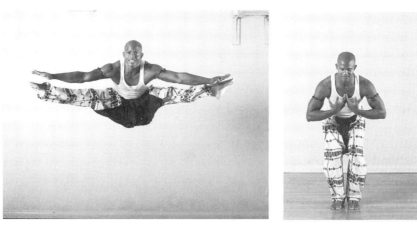

2   3

CHAPTER 13

THE JONEEBA! DANCES

TIPS ON HOW TO LEARN THE STEPS

Once the various body parts are warmed up, JONEEBA shifts into second gear. While standing in one area facing the mirror, it's time to figure out the relationship between the feet, the legs and the arms and how they relate to what the head is doing. It's about full-body coordination and learning the technique of a particular dance. Simple movements are demonstrated to allow students to get their bodies working—to get that pump. Arms swing from front to back, with legs bent and feet moving side-to-side in counts of two. Once the drummers begin to play, then the dancing begins.

JONEEBA movements are built on a pyramid structure, just as the great pyramids of Egypt were built piece by piece. Most people are mesmerized by the sheer scale of these magnificent ancient monuments. They rise from the desert sands seemingly up to heaven, a showcase of enduring architectural wonder. And yet these incredible structures weren't built starting from the apex down. Though scientists and architects are still confounded by how ancient

Egyptians actually erected the pyramids, we do know one thing: they were built from the base up. All good architects know that the foundation of any structure is the key. If the base isn't right, then nothing else will be.

The foundation of JONEEBA lies in the feet. Our feet hold the timing and the structure for all the movements. From walking to running to leaping, our feet take us where we need to go based on the directions of the drums and the dance.

When people experience JONEEBA firsthand, the power of the drums and the intensity of the movements can be overwhelming. Anxiety makes them forget that building up to a level of proficiency in JONEEBA takes time, patience, persistence, stamina and discipline.

The pyramids weren't built in one day. It took years to erect those structures. It won't take you that long to get JONEEBA, but do remember that the foundation of your body and of the JONEEBA technique is all in the feet. So, put your feet first.

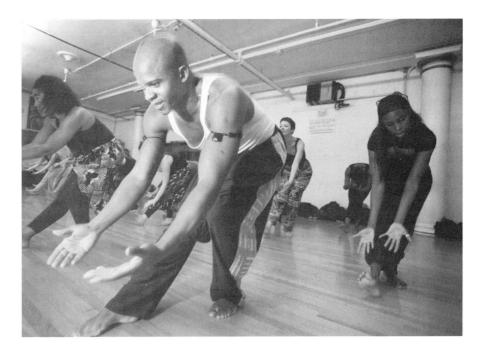

JONEEBA!

Once you get stepping with the workout, your feet will become the building blocks of your JONEEBA vocabulary. JONEEBA will provide you with the ABCs of the movements. Once you get your ABCs down, it will be time to use those fundamentals to start putting together full steps, then movements.

Did you ever diagram sentences in grammar school to learn how to write them properly? There had to be a noun and a verb in order to create a full sentence. In JONEEBA, the way to begin diagramming is through the feet. This means repeating footwork over and over until you really get it. Repetition makes the steps more solid for students.

Once you begin to understand the rhythms of the drums, you will begin to discern how the drums relate to the feet. The drums will guide your entire body and tell you the pace at which you should be dancing. The key is to watch and really listen to the drummers, whether they're in the studio or on tape.

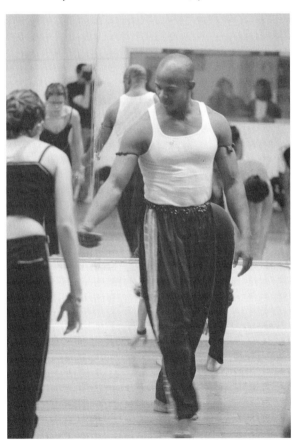

The way to make complete words and phrases in JONEEBA is to make additions with the feet. Once you are secure with the footwork of the steps, you'll move up and add the arm movements. The arms are extensions of the movements of the feet and add breadth to the dance steps. They help to give a roundness to all the movements. The arms can work in

The JONEEBA! Dances

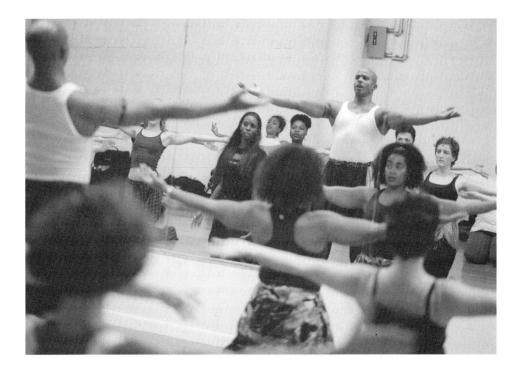

opposition to what the feet are doing, or they can work in unison with them.

Take walking, for example. I don't know anyone who walks down the street right arm swinging forward as the right foot steps ahead. On the contrary. When the right arm is in front, then the left foot initiates walking. It's just that simple. Most of us never even think twice about the fact that we walk in opposition. It's just natural, no thought process involved.

Remember that JONEEBA is also natural movement that the body will take to easily if you open your mind and let it happen using the building blocks of the dance.

Just because you've got the feet and arm movements doesn't mean that you've got the steps completely. Now it's time to add on head movements for emphasis. Rocking your head back and forth, or looking right and left or even bobbing it back to a fast steady beat all add accents to the steps.

And last but not least is the nuance of the dance step. Nuance is the overall flavor of the movement. It can be the hardest part of a dance to master because of a general perception that ethnic dance has no technique—that ethnic dance is just a lot of jumping and flailing the body around to the beat.

Nuance is about fine-tuning a movement. One dance step might have the feet stepping right, then left, with the arms swinging out and then back to the center of the body to clap. The head is bouncing in a gentle nod. Here, the nuance of the upper body is to pulse in a constant rhythm.

The point is that the nuance can be cool or hot, aggressive or sensual, light or heavy. The nuance imparts the totality of the step's feel. It is the reason you are doing a particular step quickly or slowly, with all your energy or as a time step.

Now that you've got the building blocks of JONEEBA, it's time to start dancing!

Within the limit that this book provides, I can teach you only a few steps per dance, although there are still many other steps for each of the dances. You will have an opportunity to learn both longer routines with more steps for each dance and other styles of dances from other tribes, such as sabar, kutiro and bugarabu in my advanced videos.

The name, origin and interpretation of the dance steps and music were taught to me at their sources of origin in Africa by master teachers, choreographers and musicians, who learned from their master teachers. You will find that the name, origin and interpretations may differ slightly from teacher to teacher.

SOUKOUS

THE DANCE

Sensual is the best word to describe Soukous. Hailing from Zaire and the Congo, Soukous is probably Africa's most popular music and dance style. In clubs all across the Continent, Soukous is the music that will get the crowd dancing. The word soukous, taken from the French word "soucre," means "to shake." Popularized by Africans like Franco, Pepe Kelle and Tabu Ley Rochereau, Soukous is guitar-based band music. When those sweet melodies play, the hips start to shake and roll.

SOUKOUS: Step 1

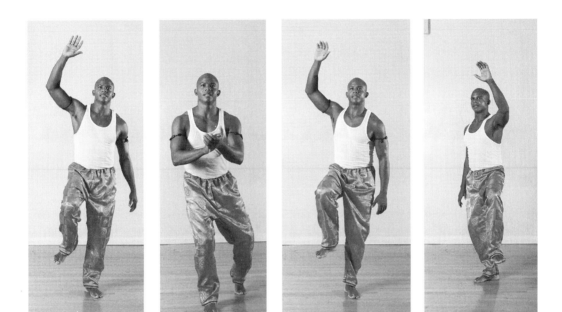

SK 1.1—Stand on left foot and lift right knee. Raise right arm overhead.

SK 1.2—Step forward on right foot and clap hands twice in front of chest.

SK 1.3—Lift right knee and raise right arm overhead.

SK 1.4—Step back on right foot and drop right arm. Raise left foot and left arm overhead.

Do the entire sequence 4x

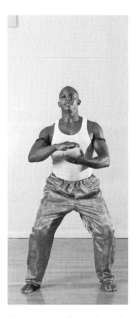

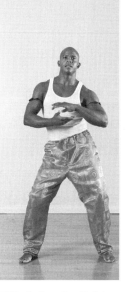

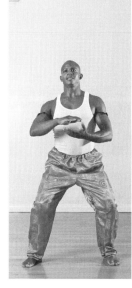

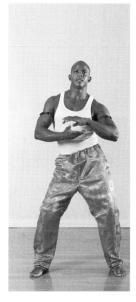

SK 2.1—Stand with feet parallel in an open second position with knees bent. Bend the arms in front of torso, with right hand over left hand. Roll hips twice, circling right, front, left and back.

SK 2.2—Roll hips twice, circling to the right (right, front, left, back) as in SK 2.1, but with left hand over right hand.

SK 2.3—Stand with feet parallel in an open second position with knees bent. Bend the arms in front of torso, with right hand over left hand. Roll hips twice, circling right, front, left and back.

SK 2.4—Roll hips twice, circling to the right (right, front, left, back) as in SK 2.1, but with left hand over right hand.

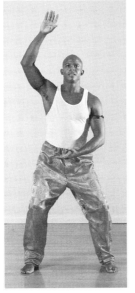 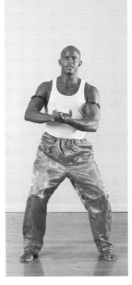 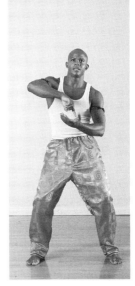

SK 2.5—Raise right arm overhead to clap hands together.

SK 2.6—Clap hands together.

SK 2.7—Roll hips in a circle to the right while circling left hand with right hand.

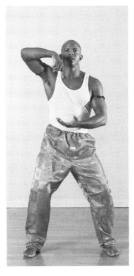 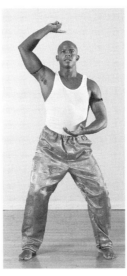 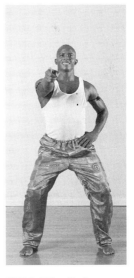

SK 2.8—Keep rolling hips and raise arm higher.

SK 2.9—Keep rolling hips, raising arm overhead.

SK 2.10—Point your right finger front contracting hips to the front with accentuation

The JONEEBA! Dances

SOUNOU

THE DANCE

This joyous West African Dance includes a lot of rocking movements. The steps are steady and soothing, done to an easy-going rhythm from the drums. The dance is said to have originated in the ancient Mali Empire. Sounou is performed to mark various celebrations.

SOUNOU: Step 1

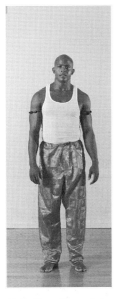

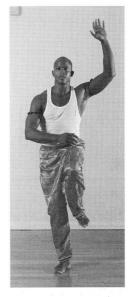

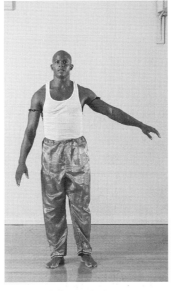

S 1.1—Stand in second position with arms at sides.

S 1.2—Raise right knee and right arm overhead. Cross left arm in front of torso. Tilt head back.

S 1.3—Set right foot down and drop both arms.

S 1.4—Raise left knee and left arm overhead. Cross right arm in front of torso.

The JONEEBA! Dances

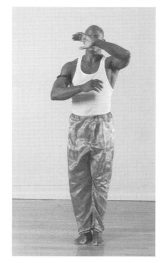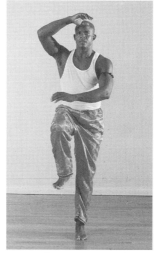

S 1.5—Set left foot down in parallel first. Bend arms in front of chest with left arm over the right.

S 1.6—Raise right knee and bent right arm overhead. Cross left arm in front of torso.

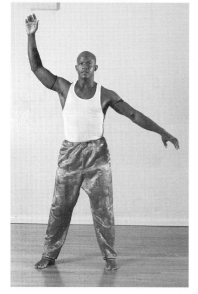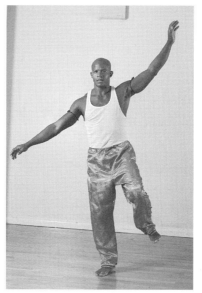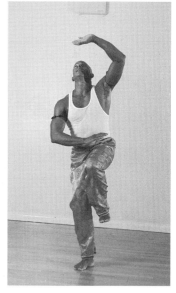

S 1.7—Lower right foot into wide second. Raise right arm and extend left arm to side.

S 1.8—Lift left foot and left arm. Extend right arm down to side.

S 1.9—Bend standing right leg and raise left knee. Lift bent left arm overhead, cross bent right arm in front of waist. Tilt head back.

JONEEBA!

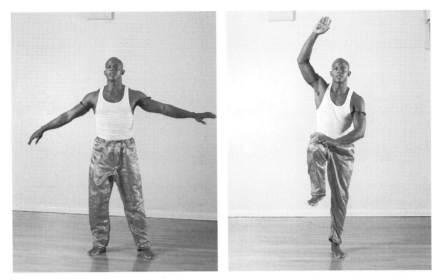

S 1.1L—Repeat S 1.1–S 1.9 on the left side. Place left foot down in second position. Swing arms to sides.

S 1. 2L—Bend standing left leg and raise right knee to step to the left together with the left foot. Lift bent right arm overhead, cross bent left arm in front of waist.

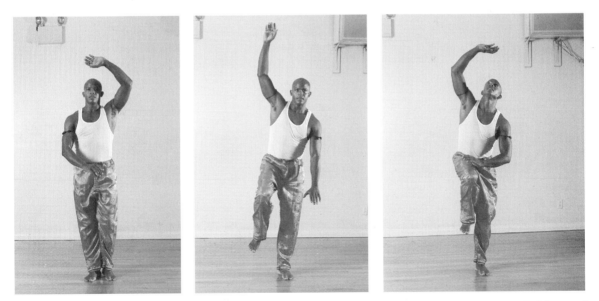

S 1.3L—Set right foot down. Lift bent left arm overhead, cross bent right arm in front of waist.

S 1.4L—Raise right knee. Lift right arm overhead and drop left arm at side.

S 1.5L—Bend standing left leg and raise right knee higher. Lift bent right arm overhead, cross bent left arm in front of waist. Tilt head back.

The JONEEBA! Dances

SOUNOU : Step 2

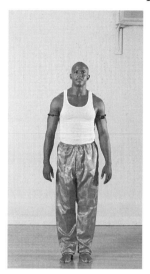

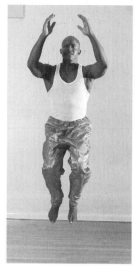

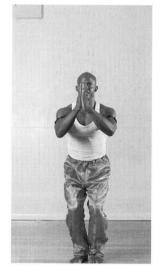

S 2.1—Stand straight up with arms at sides.

S 2.2—Jump forward with bent legs and bend both arms.

S 2.3—Land with feet together in parallel first position and bend knees. Clap hands with bent arms in front of face.

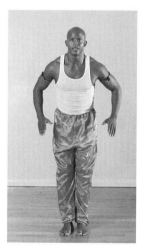

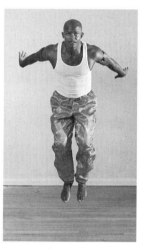

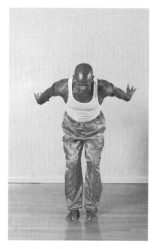

S 2.4—Straighten legs and swing hands down to jump back.

S 2.5—Jump back with bent legs and throw arms back.

S 2.6—Land with feet together, knees bent and torso leaning forward. Swing both arms back.

JONEEBA!

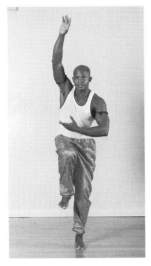 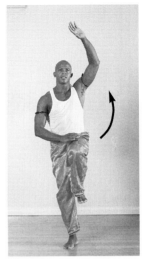

S 2.7—Lift right knee while swinging right arm overhead and left arm in front of torso.

S 2.8—Set right foot down and bend both knees. Circle right arm back down.

S 2.9—Lift left knee. Swing left arm overhead and right arm in front of torso.

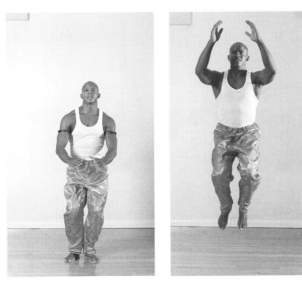

S 2.10—Set left foot down into parallel first position. Bring both arms down in front of waist.

S 2.11—Jump forward with bent legs, bending both arms.

The JONEEBA! Dances

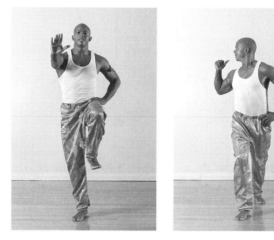

S 3.1—Stand on right foot and raise left knee. Extend right arm straight in front at shoulder level. Place left hand on left hip.

S 3.2—Reach left foot back and place on floor, bending right leg in front. Twist torso to the right and bend right arm back.

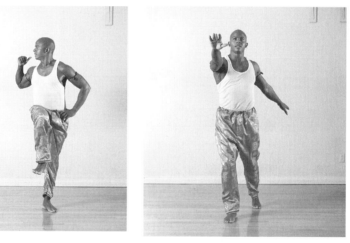

S 3.3—Stand on left foot and raise right knee.

S 3.4—Step forward on right foot and bend right knee. Extend right arm forward at shoulder level and swing left arm back.

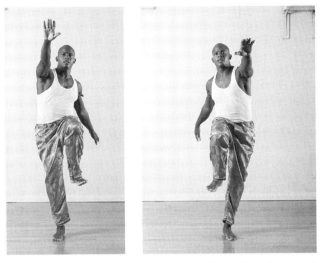

S 3.5—Lift left knee.

S 3.6—Walk on left foot and raise right knee. Extend left arm forward at shoulder level and swing right arm back.

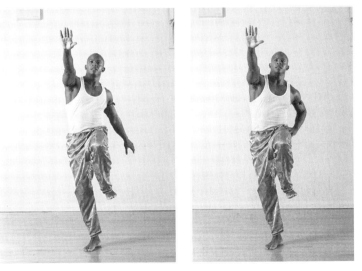

S 3.7—Jump on right foot and raise left knee. Extend right arm forward at shoulder level and swing left arm back.

S 3.8—Put left hand on hip to get into position to repeat the step from S 3.1.

The JONEEBA! Dances

Sounou : Step 4

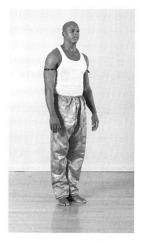 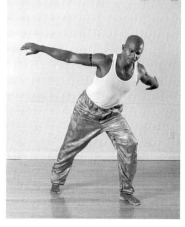 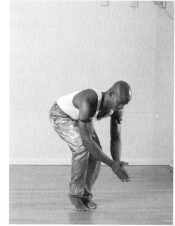

S 4.1—Start with feet together in parallel position with arms at sides.

S 4.2—Step out with left foot into lunge with left knee bent. Lean torso forward and swing arms out to sides.

S 4.3—Bring right foot forward to meet left foot in parallel position. Lean torso over the knees. Clap hands together in front of knees.

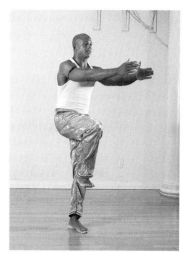 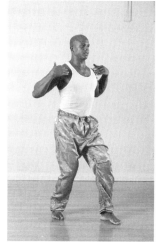 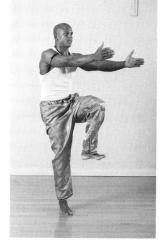

S 4.4—Lift torso and right knee. Extend both arms in front of body at shoulder level.

S 4.5—Step backwards onto right foot. Bend arms into chest at shoulders.

S 4.6—Lift left knee and extend arms in front of body at shoulder level.

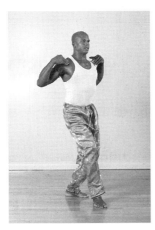 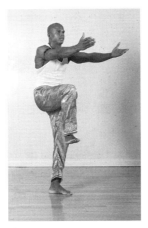 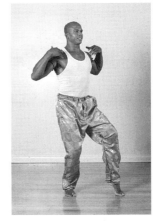

S 4.7—Step backwards onto left foot. Bend arms into chest at shoulders.

S 4.8—Lift right knee and extend arms in front of body at shoulder level.

S 4.9—Step backwards onto right foot. Bend arms into chest at shoulders.

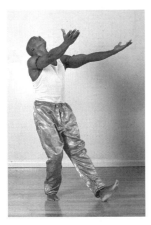 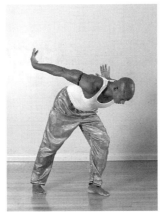 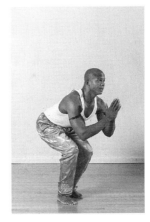

S 4.10—Extend left leg forward with left heel on floor and toes pointing up. Bend right leg. Extend arms forward with palms facing up and tilt head back.

S 4.11—Bring left foot flat on floor and lunge forward, bending left leg. Lean torso forward and swing arms back.

S 4.12—Bring right foot forward to meet left foot in parallel position while bending the knees. Lift torso slightly and bend arms in front of body with hands touching.

The JONEEBA! Dances

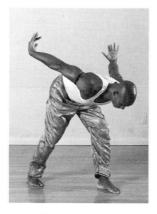 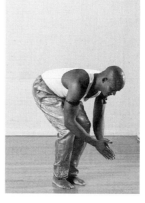

S 4.13—Lunge forward with left leg. Lean torso forward and swing arms back.

S 4.14—Bring feet into parallel first position and bend knees. Lift torso slightly and bend arms in front of body with hands touching. Repeat step from S4.4–S4.13

KOUKOU

THE DANCE

Koukou is a playful dance that is done during celebrations and parties. It is funky and fun, full of free-wheeling moves that invoke a feeling of happiness. This festive dance is said to be from Guinea, Sierra Leone and the Ivory Coast.

KOUKOU: Step 1

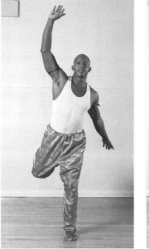

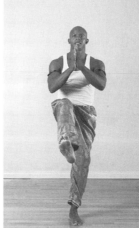

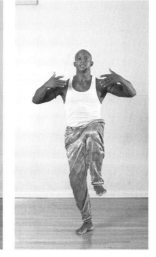

K 1.1—Swing right leg back and right arm up and left arm down.

K 1.2—Stand on left foot with right knee lifted. Hands meet in front of chest.

K 1.3—Jump back on right foot and lift left knee. Bring both hands in to shoulders.

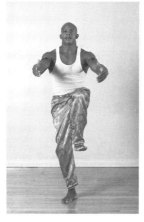

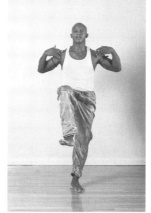

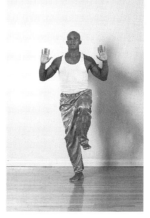

K 1.4—Extend arms over raised left knee.

K 1.5—Jump on left foot and raise right knee. Bring both hands in to shoulders.

K 1.6—Jump on right foot and raise left knee. Open arms out, with hands facing forward.

JONEEBA!

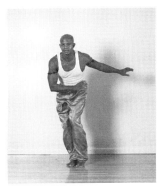

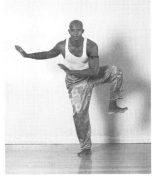

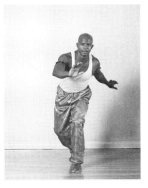

K 1.7—Bend both legs. Bend torso forward, with both arms extended to the left.

K 1.8—Lift left knee to the side, and swing both arms to the right.

K 1.9—Jump on left foot with right leg bent behind it. Reach right arm forward and swing left arm back.

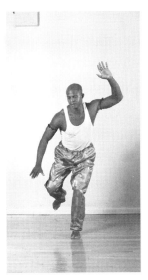

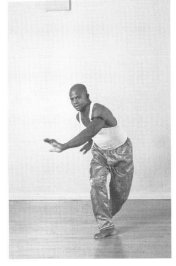

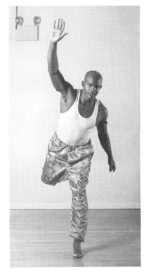

K 1.10—Shift weight to left leg and raise right foot behind it. Raise left arm and swing right arm down.

K 1.11—Jump on right foot and place left foot behind it on floor. Lean torso to the right with left arm across front of body toward right and right arm swinging back.

K 1.12—Jump on left foot with bent right leg swinging back. Raise right arm overhead and swing left arm down and start again from K 1.1.

The JONEEBA! Dances

KOUKOU: Step 2

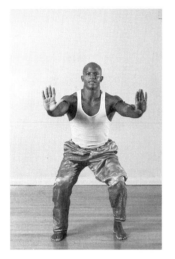

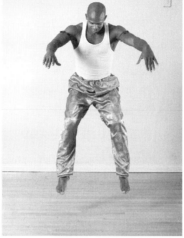

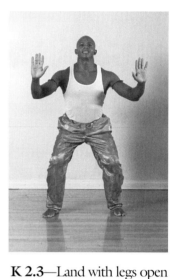

K 2.1—Jump front with legs open and parallel. Bend both legs and lean torso forward. Extend both arms forward with flexed hands.

K 2.2—Jump backward with arms forward and legs slightly bent.

K 2.3—Land with legs open and parallel. Bend torso forward and arch back and head up. Bend arms with hands facing forward.

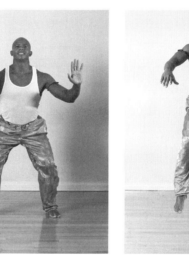

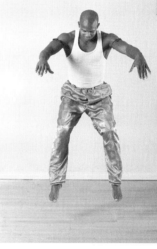

K 2.4—Jump backward with arms forward and legs slightly bent.

K 2.5—Land with legs open and parallel. Bend torso forward and arch back and head up. Bend arms with hands facing forward.

K 2.6—Jump backward with arms forward and legs slightly bent.

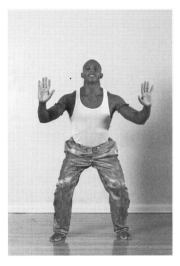 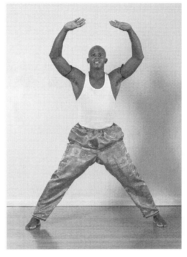 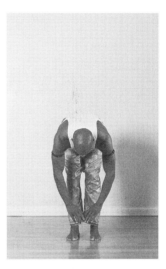

K 2.7—Land in wide second position. Bend torso forward and arch back and head up. Bend arms with hands facing forward.

K 2.8—Jump into wide second position with torso lifted and arms overhead.

K 2.9—Jump into parallel first with bent knees. Bend torso and head over knees with arms dropped and rounded over feet.

Koukou: Step 3

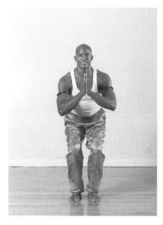

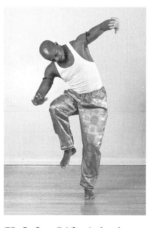

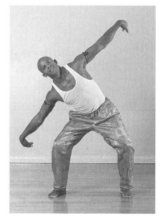

K 3.1—Lift torso and head into bent arched position. Bring hands together in front of chest.

K 3.2—Lift right knee to step open to the right. With torso leaning right, swing bent right arm toward right knee and raise bent left arm.

K 3.3—Step to the right with right foot in a wide second position with knees bent. Lean torso to right with arms and hands swinging back.

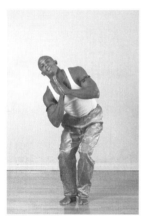

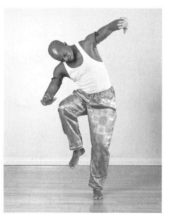

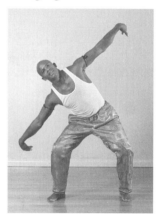

K 3.4—Bring left foot in beside right one. Bring arms in at chest with hands meeting.

K 3.5—Lift right knee to step open to the right. With torso leaning right, swing bent right arm toward right knee and raise bent left arm.

K 3.6—Step to the right with right foot in a wide second position with knees bent. Lean torso to right with arms and hands swinging back.

JONEEBA!

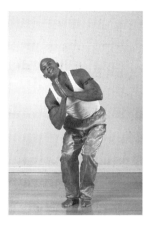

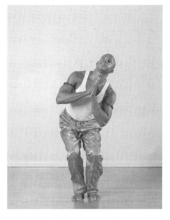

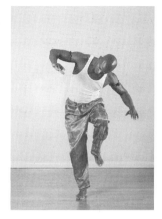

K 3.7—Bring left foot in beside right one. Bring arms in at chest with hands meeting to complete sequence.

K 3.8—Do previous sequence to the left. Arch torso and head up to the left. Bring arms in at chest with hands meeting.

K 3.9—Lift left knee to step to the left with torso leaning left, swing bent left arm toward left knee and raise bent right arm.

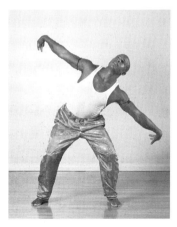

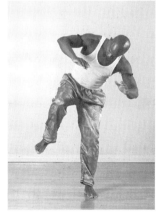

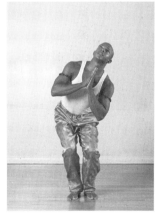

K 3.10—Step out to left side in wide second with knees bent. Lean torso to left with arms swinging back.

K 3.11—Stand on left foot and raise right knee. Bend torso forward and bend both arms in at chest.

K 3.12—Bring feet into parallel first with knees bent. Lean torso to the left. Bring arms in at chest with hands meeting.

The JONEEBA! Dances

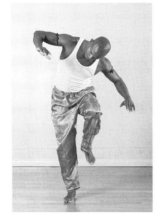

K 3.13—Stand on right foot and lift left knee. With torso leaning to left, swing bent left arm toward left knee and raise bent right arm.

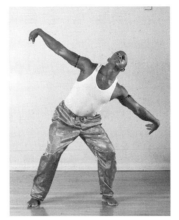

K 3.14—Step out to left side in wide second with knees bent. Lean torso to left with arms swinging back.

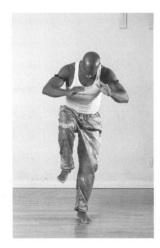

K 3.15—Stand on left foot and raise right knee. Bend torso forward and bend both arms in at chest.

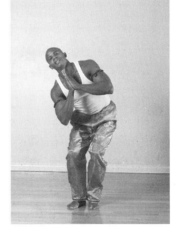

K 3.16—Bring feet into parallel first position, with knees bent. Arch torso and head up to the right. Bring arms in at chest with hands meeting to start again from K 3.2.

DOUNOUMBA

THE DANCE

Dounoumba is a dance of strength. Its movements are powerful and often acrobatic. Though both men and women perform the dance, it is clearly a showcase of male virility. The dance is from the Malinke of Guinea and Mali. The thunderous bass of the doundoun drum accentuates this dance's forceful moves.

This dance will present a seperate series of steps for ladies and men.

DOUNOUMBA: LADIES' Step 1

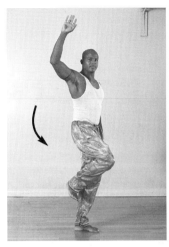
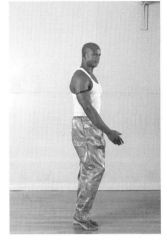
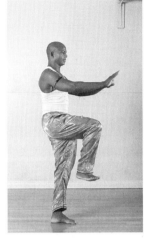

DL 1.1—Stand on left leg, with right leg bent, facing on left diagonal. Raise right arm in air. Left arm is at left side.

DL 1.2—Face left and swing your right arm down as you step on your right foot.

DL 1.3—Lift right knee and extend both arms to the front.

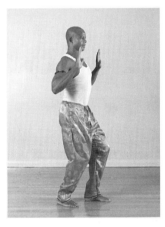
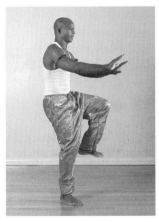
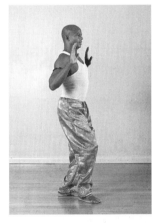

DL 1.4—Step back, placing right foot down with bent knees. Bend arms in toward shoulders.

DL 1.5—Lift left knee and extend both arms to the front.

DL 1.6—Step back, placing left foot down with bent knees. Bend arms in toward shoulders.

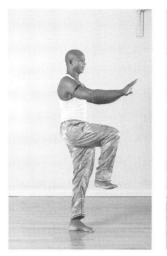 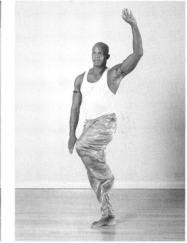

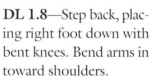

DL 1.7—Lift right knee and extend both arms to the front.

DL 1.8—Step back, placing right foot down with bent knees. Bend arms in toward shoulders.

DL 1.9—Repeat previous sequence to the left. Stand on right leg with left leg bent facing on right diagonal. Raise left arm in air, keeping it bent slightly. Right arm is at right side.

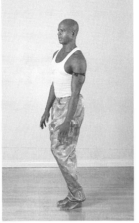
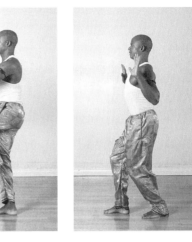

DL1.10—Face right and place left foot on floor. Bring left arm down.

DL 1.11—Lift left knee and extend both arms to the front.

DL 1.12—Step back, placing left foot down with bent knees. Bend arms in toward shoulders.

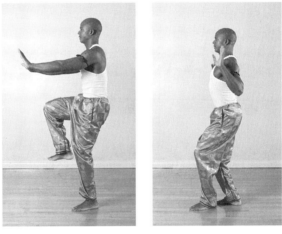

DL 1.13—Lift right knee and extend both arms to the front.

DL 1.14—Step back, placing right foot down, keeping knees bent. Bend arms in toward shoulders.

JONEEBA!

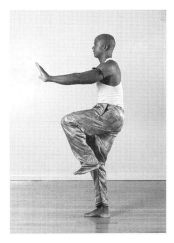 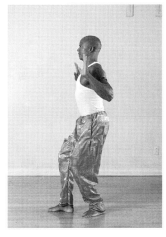

DL 1.15—Lift left knee and extend both arms to the front.

DL 1.16—Step back, setting left foot down, keeping knees bent. Bend arms in toward shoulders to start right again.

DOUNOUMBA: LADIES' STEP 2

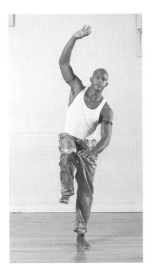

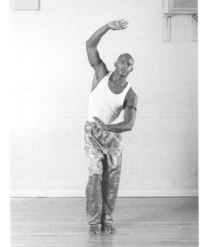

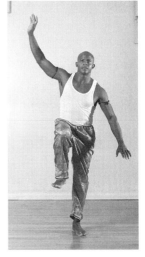

DL 2.1—Stand with right knee raised. Lift right arm overhead and bring left arm to right knee.

DL 2.2—Step left with weight on left leg and right foot on demi-point (weight on ball of foot with heel raised). Bend both legs. Raise right arm overhead and bring bent left arm in front of waist.

DL 2.3—Straighten left leg, lift right knee and right arm. Left arm falls to left side.

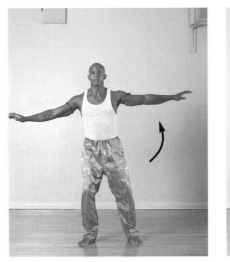

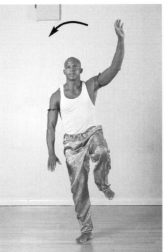

DL 2.4—Step onto right foot and swing arms out to sides.

DL 2.5—Stand on right leg, lift left knee and left arm. Right arm falls to right side.

JONEEBA!

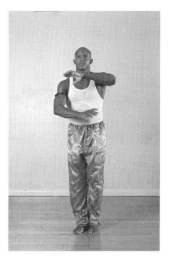

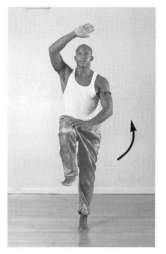

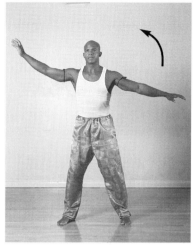

DL 2.6—Stand with legs in parallel first. Arms are bent at front of torso, with left arm over the right.

DL 2.7—Lift right knee and right arm, standing on left leg. Left arm falls toward right knee.

DL 2.8—Step onto right foot and swing arms out to sides.

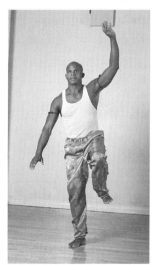

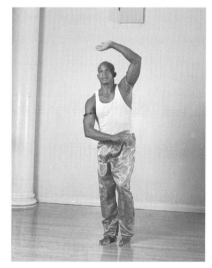

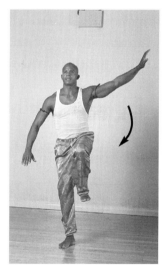

DL 2.9—Stand on right foot, lift left knee and left arm. Right arm falls to right side.

DL 2.10—Do the same step going to your left. Step right with weight on right leg, with left foot on demi-point (weight on ball of foot with heel raised). Raise left arm overhead and bring bent right arm in front of waist.

DL 2.11—Straighten right leg, lift left knee and left arm. Right arm falls to right side.

The JONEEBA! Dances

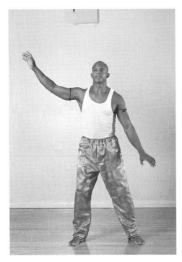

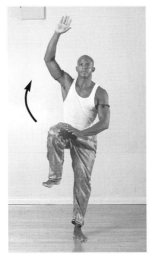

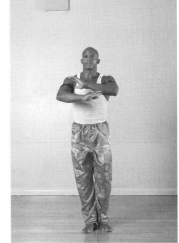

DL 2.12—Step onto left foot and swing right arm up and left arm down.

DL 2.13—Stand on left leg, lift right knee and right arm. Left arm comes to waist.

DL 2.14—Place right foot down into parallel first. Bend arms in front of chest with left arm over right arm.

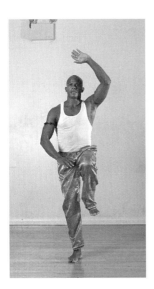

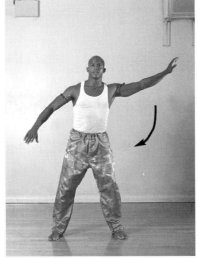

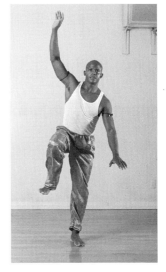

DL 2.15—Lift left knee and left arm, standing on right leg. Right arm falls toward left knee.

DL 2.16—Step onto left foot and swing arms out to sides.

DL 2.17—Lift right knee and right arm. Left arm falls to left side to start from first step (DL 2.1).

DOUNOUMBA: LADIES' STEP 3

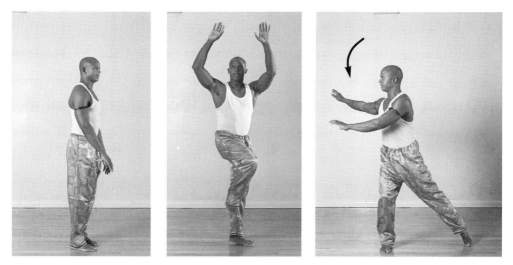

DL 3.1—Starting position: stand with feet together and parallel, facing front with arms down.

DL 3.2—Lift right knee and raise arms overhead to step back onto right foot.

DL 3.3—Step to the back on the right foot with right knee bent. Left leg remains to the front. Arms swing from the right side to the back.

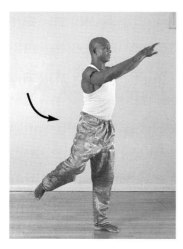

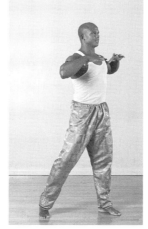

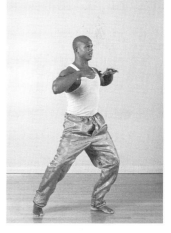

DL 3.4—Step forward onto left foot preparing to step onto right foot. Both arms swing to the front at eye level.

DL 3.5—Step onto right foot. Bring arms in, bending at shoulders.

DL 3.6—Shake your chest as you bend your left knee while keeping your hands touching your chest.

The JONEEBA! Dances

Dounoumba: Ladies' Step 4

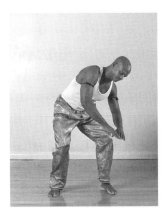

DL 4.1—Bend both legs. Bend torso over toward left leg, with hands meeting at left knee.

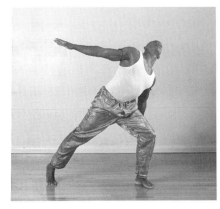

DL 4.2—Step left with left knee bent facing left side and right leg extended back diagonally. Swing right arm front, up and back. Left arm swings down and back. Head should tilt back.

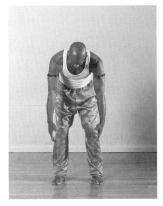

DL 4.3—Bring right foot together parallel with the left foot while bending knees. Torso is bent over, with arms hanging toward the floor.

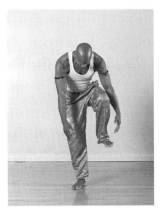

DL 4.4—Lift left foot. Bend torso forward and drop arms down toward left foot.

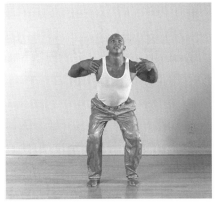

DL 4.5—Place left foot down with knees bent. Bring hands toward shoulders while arching your head and back. Keep your torso bent forward.

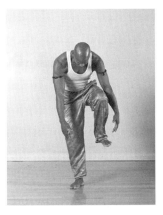

DL 4.6—Lift left foot. Bend torso forward and drop arms down toward left foot.

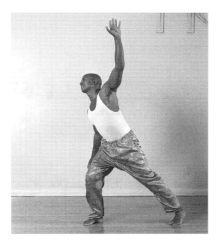

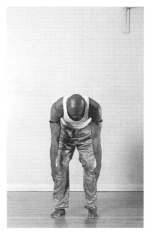

DL 4.7—Repeat previous sequence to the left. Step back onto left foot with right knee bent in front on a diagonal and left leg extended back diagonally. Left arm swings front, up and back. Right arm swings down and back. Head tilts back.

DL 4.8—Bring left foot parallel with right foot while bending knees. Torso is bent over, with arms hanging toward the floor.

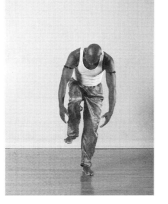

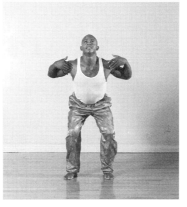

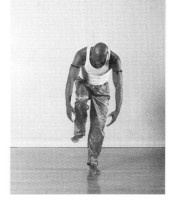

DL 4.9—Lift right foot. Bend torso forward and drop arms down toward left foot.

DL 4.10—Place right foot down with knees bent. Bring hands toward shoulders with back and head arching back while keeping the torso bent forward.

DL 4.11—Lift right foot. Bend torso forward and drop arms down toward left foot to start again with right leg extended back. (DL 4.2)

The JONEEBA! Dances

DOUNOUMBA: MEN'S STEP 1

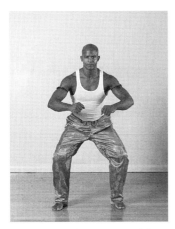

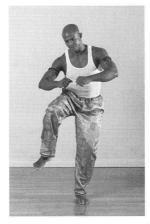

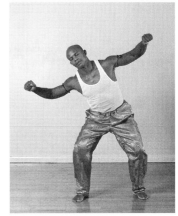

DM 1.1—Starting position: stand with feet wide and knees bent. Lean torso forward, bringing bent arms toward chest with hands in front of chest.

DM 1.2—Lift right knee, leaning to right.

DM 1.3—Set right foot down. Lean torso more to the right with arms bent out to sides.

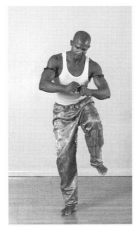

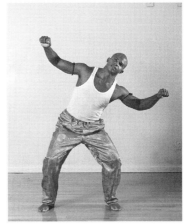

DM 1.4—Lift left knee, leaning to left.

DM 1.5—Place left foot down. Lean torso more to the left with arms bent out to sides. Repeat DM 1.2–DM 1.5.

DOUNOUMBA: MEN's Step 2 (Same sequence as Ladies' Step 2)

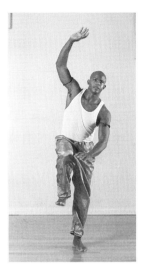

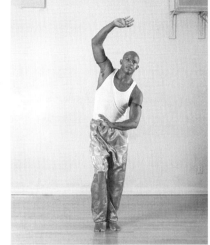

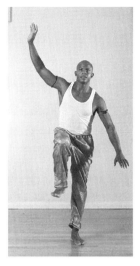

DM 2.1—Stand with right knee raised. Lift right arm overhead and bring left arm to right knee.

DM 2.2—Stand with weight on left leg with right foot on demi-point (weight on ball of foot with heel raised). Bend both legs. Raise right arm overhead and bring bent left arm in front of waist.

DM 2.3—Straighten left leg, lift right knee and right arm. Left arm falls to left side.

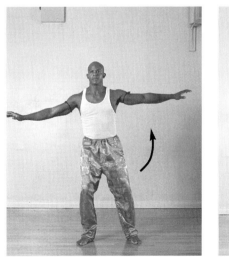

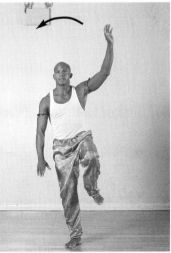

DM 2.4—Step onto right foot and swing arms out to sides.

DM 2.5—Stand on right leg, lift left knee and left arm. Right arm falls to right side.

The JONEEBA! Dances

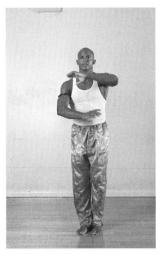

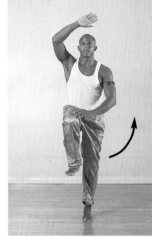

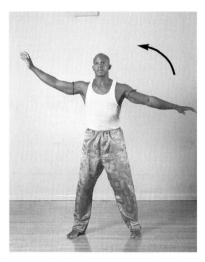

DM 2.6—Stand with legs in parallel first. Arms are bent at front of torso, with left arm over the right.

DM 2.7—Lift right knee and right arm, standing on left leg. Left arm falls toward right knee.

DM 2.8—Step onto right foot and swing arms out to sides.

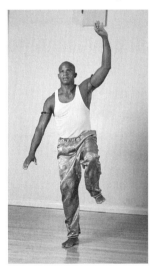

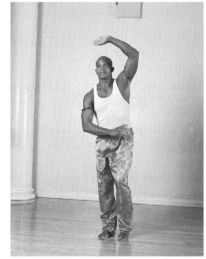

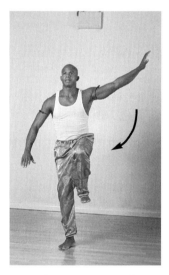

DM 2.9—Stand on right foot, lift left knee and left arm. Right arm falls to right side.

DM 2.10—Do the same step going to your left. Stand with weight on right leg, with left foot on demi-point (weight on ball of foot with heel raised). Raise left arm overhead and bring bent right arm in front of waist.

DM 2.11—Straighten right leg, lift left knee and left arm. Right arm falls to right side.

JONEEBA!

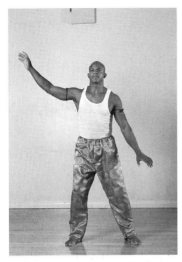

DM 2.12—Step onto left foot and swing right arm up and left arm down.

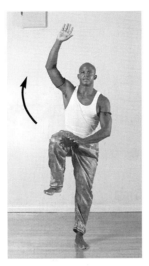

DM 2.13—Stand on left leg, lift right knee and right arm. Left arm comes to waist.

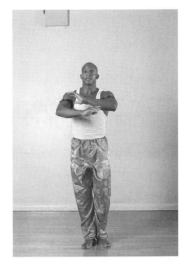

DM 2.14—Place right foot down into parallel first. Bend arms in front of chest with left arm over right arm.

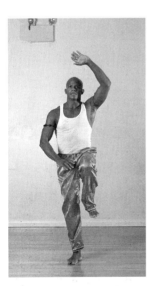

DM 2.15—Lift left knee and left arm, standing on right leg. Right arm falls toward left knee.

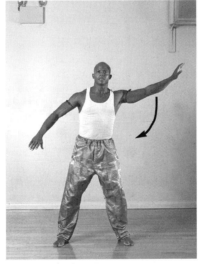

DM 2.16—Step onto left foot and swing arms out to sides.

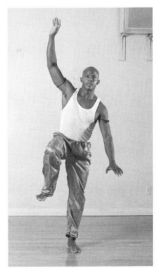

DM 2.17—Lift right knee and right arm. Left arm falls to left side to start from first step (DM 2.1).

The JONEEBA! Dances

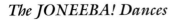

DOUNOUMBA: MEN's Step 3

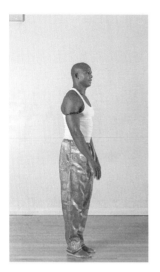

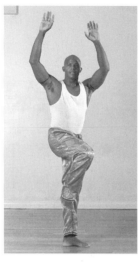

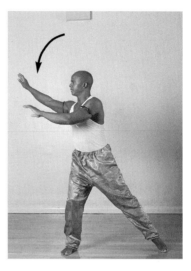

DM 3.1—Starting position: stand with feet together and parallel, facing front with arms down.

DM 3.2—Raise right knee, and raise arms overhead. Torso faces front.

DM 3.3—Jump to right into a lunge, with right knee bent and left leg straight to side. Both arms swing to right.

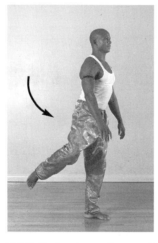

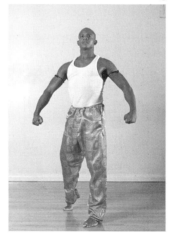

DM 3.4—Step forward onto left foot. Both arms should drop to the front at waist level.

DM 3.5—Right foot is in a demi-point behind. Torso is upright with arms pushed out, and hands are clenched.

DOUNOUMBA: MEN'S STEP 4

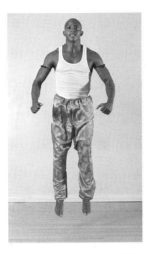 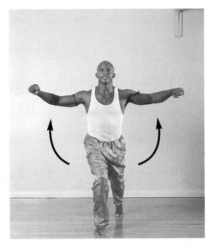 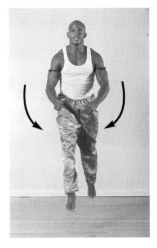

DM 4.1—Jump straight up with arms down and hands in fists.

DM 4.2—Land on both feet at the same time, with right knee bent forward. Bent arms and elbows swing upward on the landing to accent the fall. The torso should be upright to accent the front.

DM 4.3—Jump straight up with arms down, hands in fists, and right foot front.

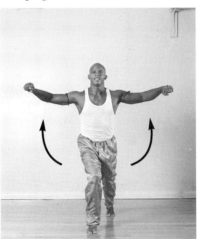

DM 4.4—Land on both feet at the same time, with right knee bent forward. Bent arms and elbows swing upward on the landing to accent the fall. The torso should be upright to accent the front.

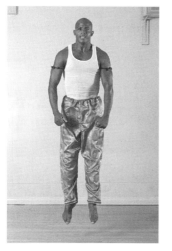

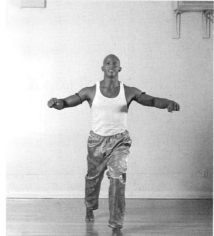

DM 4.5—Jump straight up with arms down and hands in fists.

DM 4.6—Land on both feet at the same time, with left knee bent forward. Bent arms and elbows swing upward on the landing to accent the fall. The torso should be upright to accent the front.

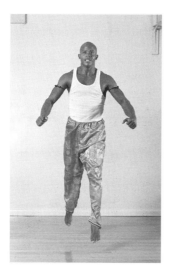

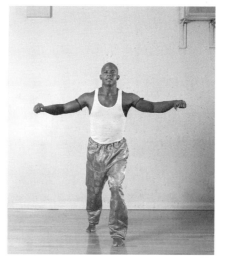

DM 4.7—Jump straight up with arms down, hands in fists, and left foot front.

DM 4.8—Land on both feet at the same time, with left knee bent forward. Bent arms and elbows swing upward on the landing to accent the fall. The torso should be upright to accent the front. Start again from DM 4.1.

JONEEBA!

MANJIANI

The Dance

Manjiani is a high-energy, fast-paced dance done in West Africa. Its moves are dynamic and challenging. This social dance is performed during celebrations. It is said that Manjiani had been danced in earlier generations by young girls. The drumming is intense and quick to match the speed of the movements.

MANJIANI: Step 1

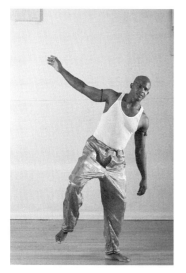

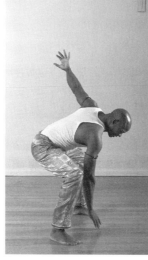

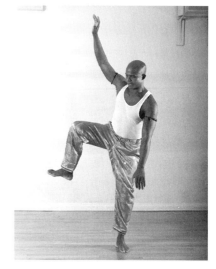

M 1.1—Hop onto left foot, lifting right foot. Lean torso to the left and lift right arm up, keeping left arm down.

M 1.2—Step forward onto right foot and throw torso and right arm forward. Left arm swings back.

M 1.3—Bring right foot back with a hop onto left foot. Lift torso. Right knee and right arm should be up. Left arm falls to the side.

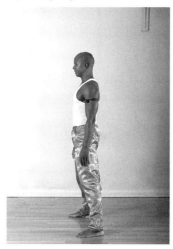

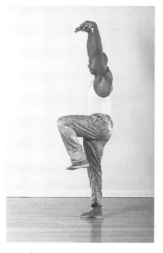

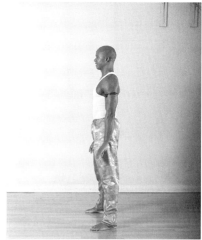

M 1.4—Step back onto right foot and face right. Drop both arms to sides.

M 1.5—Lift left knee and raise both arms overhead.

M 1.6—Stomp down with left foot and drop both arms to sides to accent the move.

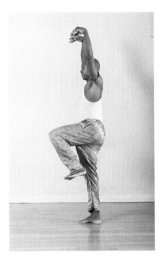

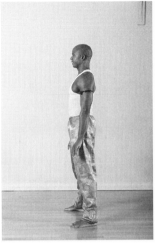

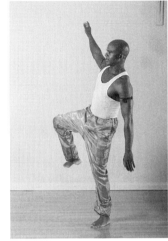

M 1.7—Lift left knee and raise both arms overhead a second time.

M 1.8—Stomp down with left foot and drop both arms to sides a second time.

M 1.9—Lift right foot and lean torso to the left. Swing right arm up, keeping left arm down to start again from M 1.2.

The JONEEBA! Dances

MANJIANI: Step 2

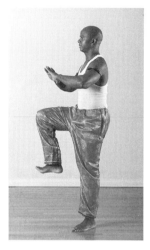

M 2.1—Face right side. Raise right knee and bend arms into chest.

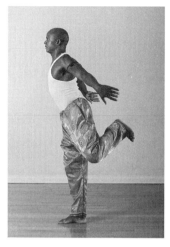

M 2.2—Jump onto right foot and raise bent left leg. Swing both arms to the back.

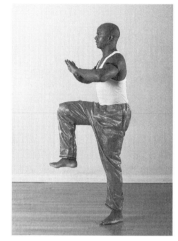

M 2.3—Jump onto left foot, raising right knee. Bend arms into chest.

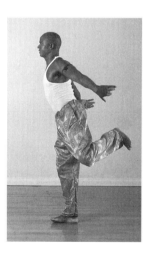

M 2.4—Jump onto right foot and raise bent left leg. Swing both arms to the back.

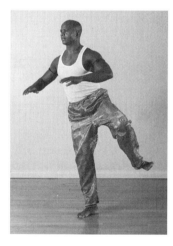

M 2.5—Shift weight on right leg to face center with left knee lifted. Bring both arms to your chest.

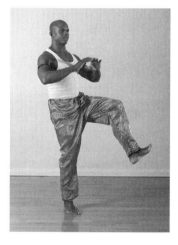

M 2.6—Turn to left side, with left knee raised. Bend arms into chest.

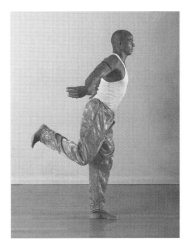

M 2.7—Jump onto left foot and raise bent right leg. Swing both arms to the back.

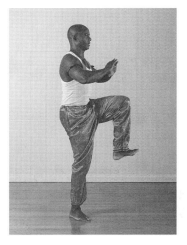

M 2.8—Jump onto right foot and raise left knee. Bend arms into chest.

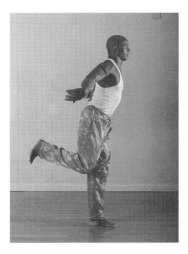

M 2.9—Jump onto left foot and raise bent right leg. Swing both arms to the back.

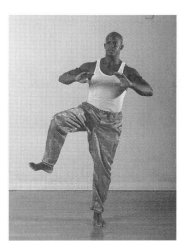

M 2.10—Shift weight on left leg to face center with right knee lifted. Bend arms into chest to start from M 2.1.

MANJIANI: Step 3

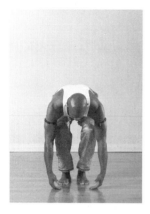

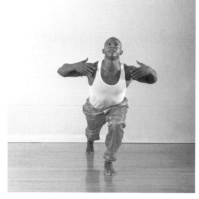

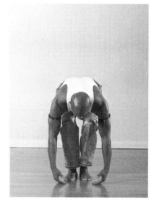

M 3.1—Place feet in parallel first position and bend knees. Bend torso, head and arms over knees.

M 3.2—Step back with right foot, extending the leg back. Left foot is forward. Arch torso and head up. Lift bent arms up and bring your hands to meet shoulders.

M 3.3—Bring right foot forward to meet left foot back in starting position (M 3.1).

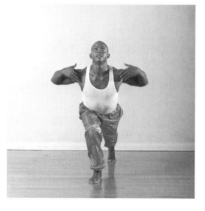

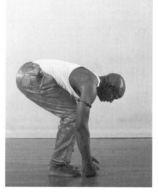

M 3.4—Step back with left foot, extending the leg back. Right foot is forward. Arch torso and head up. Lift bent arms up and bring your hands to meet shoulders.

M 3.5—Bring left foot forward to meet right foot, and start again from M 3.1.

Now You Have Learned the Basics!

CHAPTER 14

ENDING THE CLASS

THE CIRCLE

So, you've completed your warm-up and the dances, but the drummers just won't stop. Well, guess what? It's time to form a circle around the drummers

and express yourself, your individuality . . . your unique
style and movement. It's the
ultimate time for getting
your spirit in powerful harmony and connection with
the dance, the drummers
and the music.

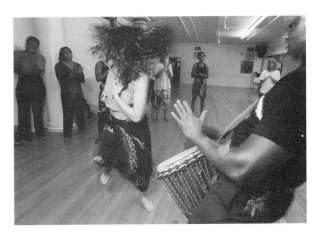

The circle should be
open and the community of
dancers (if you are in a dance
studio, or dancing with a

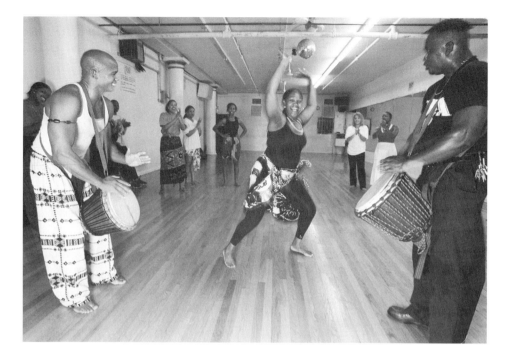

group of friends) and drummers positive. Anyone who wants to join the circle should be able to. As each dancer comes out to do his or her thing, a friendly competition emerges. The competition is not about who does the fanciest footwork, but about how the community of students can dance to take the energy in the class higher and higher. It's about fun. Some people jump out into the circle and act silly. Others get out there and do whatever they feel inside. Then there are those who will do the steps I've just taught in class. They are getting connected to their true selves, and everybody has fun watching them because they're having such a good time.

In Senegal, there was one guy who would always come into the sabar circle. The thing that was amazing about him was that whenever he was there he was not even doing sabar! But everybody cheered him on and loved to see him dance. Why? Because he let the rhythm of the drums free him. The JONEEBA circle is about energy and letting the body tap into the spirit freely. It's not about technical proficiency in a particular dance. The people watching and the drummers become united spiritually with the person who is having a great time dancing because that person's energy and spirit is free.

The upshot of all this energy is a feeling of freedom and joy. Dancers have gotten a chance to express who they are through the dance and the community and go away feeling uplifted. The movement and the music get rid of inertia and heaviness, and a sense of lightness and joy move in. The entire experience ends up being therapeutic for all involved. In fact, I have even had students tell me that since they started taking JONEEBA classes, they no longer go see their therapists! The dance and the drum have brought their spirits back and their lives feels complete because they're in harmony with their inner selves.

In my class, everyone positive is welcome. Africans, Europeans, Asians, Latinos, professionals and blue-collar workers dance, drum, laugh and communicate on a common level—as human beings.

I have found that JONEEBA students and musicians are a group of people who are open-minded, free and down-to-earth.

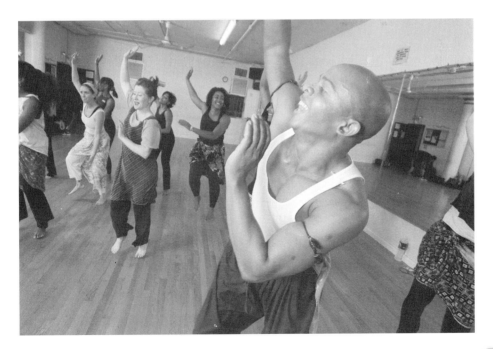

They are people sharing a beautiful art form and who respect each other and have fun together in a positive and healthy environment. You too will feel welcome. This is an amazing journey of freedom.

HOW TO JOIN THE CIRCLE

Do not be concerned about people watching you or about messing up. Fear is only natural. My advice is to think of going into the circle as if you are going to cleanse and heal yourself, as if you have to go. Definitely don't try to impress anybody or show off. Dance for yourself. The first time, pick only one step to dance. Of course, if you want to do more, that's fine, too. You can use a step done in class or any move that you know. As you become more experienced you can do more than one step. Smile and have fun!

Those of you who are doing my workout at home will experience the same type of joy, but in a different way. You will feel the oneness as you listen to the recordings of musicians playing the drums, and you also will see an improvement in your body as well as in your spirit—an absolutely wonderful workout.

Go ahead, turn up the CD or the cassette player and let your spirit run free. That's what JONEEBA time is all about.

COOLING DOWN:

After you've finished participating in the circle of your JONEEBA class, I suggest that you do some additional stretching exercises. They will help to increase the length of tight and poorly functioning muscles, decrease any soreness and maintain healthy muscles.

JONEEBA! CERTIFICATIONS

Are you enjoying your JONEEBA workout? If you are and you don't live in New York, or if you are doing this workout by yourself but would like to work out with a group in your area, why not become a JONEEBA certified instructor? It's easy. First, see if you can get an informal group together. You know, some people who are fun to be around who want to get in shape and are searching for that inner joy and peace . . . well, you know what you've gotten from these workouts. Let's see, perhaps some members of your family, friends, or co-workers. Now, you're ready to start your own class. You can become a certified JONEEBA instructor. Only certified JONEEBA instructors are allowed to teach JONEEBA classes. So, if you've found your rhythm, follow your spirit. (See the back of the book for more information.)

ABOUT THE AUTHOR

A. Djoniba Mouflet is the creator of JONEEBA, the African dance work-out. Thousands of people have waited in line to attend his dynamic classes at the Manhattan-based Djoniba Dance and Drum Centre.

From a poverty-ridden childhood in Martinique to sleeping on the subway in New York City, Djoniba has overcome a myriad of obstacles through sheer spirit of determination. Today, the multilingual, multi-talented Djoniba is widely recognized and respected as a shrewd businessman as well as an ac-claimed dancer/choreographer, performer and one of the finest drum com-posers and master teachers internationally. He's also adept in ballet, jazz and modern dance. Since he began teaching African dance and drumming 16 years ago, and later the JONEEBA technique, he has become a veritable dance in-stitution worldwide.

Djoniba studied dance, drum and music in Senegal, Guinea and Mali in West Africa. In addition to attending Mudra Afrique Center of Perfectionism and Research of West African Arts, a performing arts school, he also studied with the Ballet Foret Sacre, Ballet Meissa, Ballet Conakry and the National

Ballets African of Guinea. His teachers included such traditional masters as Ousman Seck, Josy Michalon, Jean Claude Lamorandiere, Doudou N'Diaye Rose, Bouly Sankho, Cheick Niang, Tapha Cisse, Arafan and Kemoko Sano, Ahmidou Bangoura and Germaine Acogny. In 1982, Djoniba moved to New York, where Arthur Mitchell, founder of the Dance Theater of Harlem, awarded him a scholarship to study at the prestigious school. In 1994, Djoniba opened the Djoniba Dance and Drum Centre, located off Park Avenue in the heart of New York City.

Today, the school is credited as the largest ethnic-based dance and drum schools in the world. Here, Djoniba has taught his JONEEBA technique to thousands of students. In addition, he also has taught as well as performed throughout the world, including many countries in Africa, Europe, Asia and North and South America, as well as places such as Walt Disney World and Busch Gardens. He also has worked with a variety of artists, including singer Chaka Khan and filmmaker Spike Lee.

In 1990, A. Djoniba Mouflet founded Ballet D'Afrique, a company of dancers and musicians who strive to share with their audiences the power and mysticism of traditional West African dance and music. With Djoniba's intricate choreography, staging and powerful music composition, the company was an instant success. Dazzling fire eaters, intriguing masks and breath-taking acrobat-stilt walkers transported many audiences to the vibrant world of West African music and dance in a journey delighting the soul and senses.

Their extensive international touring have included performances on some of the most prestigious stages around the world, museums across the United States (Guggenheim Museum, Museum of Natural History, etc.), hundreds of public schools in New York and New Jersey and more.

Djoniba has contributed greatly to the introduction and expansion of African dance and music in the U.S., resulting in greater visibility for African artists and African music and dance as a whole.

For the past ten years, he has exposed hundreds of Caucasians, Asians and Blacks of all ages to the beauty and richness of African culture through his annual cultural exchange trips to Africa during the summer months.

In addition, the annual three-day Djoniba Dance and Drum Festival is yet another vehicle Djoniba utilizes to showcase African culture, and at the same time, honor outstanding artists such as the legendary dancer/choreographer and multi-talented artist Geoffrey Holder for their contributions to the world of dance.

Djoniba is also the founder of the highly inspirational and motivational program, the Djoniba Dance and Drum Kids. This multi-cultural program is geared for children ages 3–16 to study and perform dance, drum, ballet and capoeira. At the heart of this program is Djoniba's commitment to provide scholarships or reduced tuition for students from low-income families.

This effort is Djoniba's way of "giving back" to the worldwide community. In the same way that God has opened the universe to embrace and provide for him, Djoniba fully and graciously is giving back. Over the past six years, he has given his talent, time and finances to provide more than 500 young students with an opportunity to study dance and drumming, which helps to build their self-esteem and confidence for a brighter future.

A. Djoniba Mouflet has come a long way. He is an illustrious example of JONEEBA: spirit, mind and body working in harmony to accomplish all he was placed on earth to be and to do. Djoniba is a model and example for many whose lives he has inspired and changed. He is a man who follows his spirit.

GLOSSARY

JONEEBA Terms

Balaphon: Wooden instrument similar to the modern xylophone.

Break: Musical phrase that signals a change in movement or rhythm.

Bugarabu: Dance/music from South Senegal (Casamance, from the Djola Tribe).

Chaya: Loose-fitting pants traditionally worn by men.

Conga: Barrel-shaped drum of Afro-Cuban origin that is played with the hands.

Djimbe: Goblet-shaped drum played with the hands. Originated in the Mali Empire, it is played throughout Africa.

Djimbefola: Master djimbe player.

Doundoun: Large two-headed drum made of wood or a metal container. Played with sticks.

Dounounba: Dance of strength from the Malinke of Mali and Guinea.

Griot: Musician, singer or oral historian whose stories and praises relate to cultural history.

Kenkeni: Small two-headed drum played with sticks.

Kora: Harp/lute with 21 strings often played by Malinke griots.

Koukou: Playful social dance said to be from Guinea, Sierra Leone and Ivory Coast.

Kutiro: Dance/drums from South Senegal (Casamance, from the Djola Tribe).

Lapa: Traditional wrap worn by women in Africa, similar to a sarong.

Manding: Ethnic group in West Africa also known as Malinke, Mandingo, Mandinka, Bambara or Djoula (tradesmen).

Manjiani: High-energy dance done in West Africa.

M'Balax: Senegalese pop music.

Sabar: Family of drums and dance style from the Wolof people of Senegal.

Salsa: Pop music and dance style from Latin America.

Samba: Popular Brazilian dance and music with roots in south-west Africa.

Shekere: Large gourd rattle.

Songba/Songbeni: Medium-size two-headed drum played with sticks.

Glossary

Soukous: Congolese pop music.

Sounou: West African dance said to have originated in Mali Empire.
Tanabere: Senegalese block party with sabar dancing and drumming.

Zouk: Caribbean pop music from Martinique.

Names and Places

Les Ballets Africains de Keita Fodeba: Company founded in
  Paris in 1952 by Keita Fodeba, the godfather of staged African
  dance.

Les Ballet Africains de Guinea: National dance company of
  Guinea founded in the 1960s.

Mali Empire: One of the largest, most powerful empires in Africa
  that rose to power under Sundiata Keita in 1235 A.D. The empire included parts of present-day Mali, Guinea, Niger, Burkino
  Faso, Guinea-Bissau, Mauritania, Senegal and Gambia.

Sekou Toure: First president of Guinea after it gained independence in 1958.

Master West African drummers:
  Doudou N'Diaye Rose (Senegal)
  Ladji Camara (Guinea)
  Babatunde Olatunji (Nigeria)
  Tapha Cisse (Senegal)
  Arona N'Diaye Rose (Senegal)

Master West African dancers/choreographers:
  Ousman Seck (Senegal)
  Kemoko Sano (Guinea)

JONEEBA!

SELECTED BIBLIOGRAPHY

Research on the Mali Empire in the Middle Ages, Djibril Tamsir Niane.

Liberte Negritude et Humanisme, Leopold Sedar Senghor.

The Music of Africa, J.H. Kwabena Nketia, W.W. Norton & Co., 1974.

African Music: A People's Art, Francis Bebey, Lawrence Hill Books, 1975.

Mandiani Drum and Dance: Djimbe Performance and Black Aesthetics from Africa to the New World, Mark Sunkett, White Cliffs Media Inc., 1995.

The Drummer's Path: Moving the Spirit with Ritual and Traditional Drumming, Sule Greg Wilson, Destiny Books, 1992.

Africa O-Ye!: A Celebration of African Music, Graeme Ewens, Da Capo Press Inc., 1991.

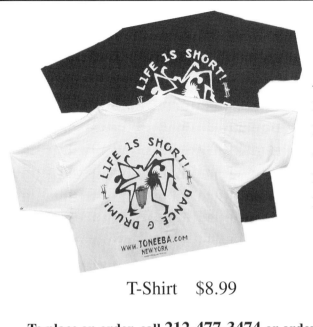
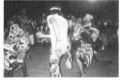
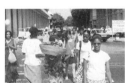

JONEEBA TEACHER CERTIFICATION

- Become a qualified and certified JONEEBA teacher and teach in gyms, health clubs, and schools!

- Learn how to teach and relate to your students

- Learn principles of exercise and nutrition

- Learn basic injury prevention

- Learn how to maximize your workout

- Learn how to play basic rhythms on the drums, and more!

Call for more details, course description, prices and dates.
212-477-3474 or www.Joneeba.com

The CD "Drums for Your Soul"

Captivating drumming rhythms, and music for your JONEEBA class and listening pleasure.

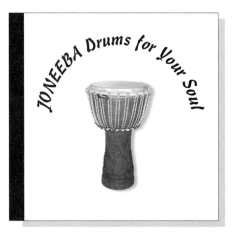

www.Joneeba.com or 212-477-3474